Reimagining the Frozen Banana

Scrumptious and Healthy Recipes with Frozen Bananas

Joshua Millstein
Illustrated by Amit Millstein

Reimagining the Frozen Banana

Reimagining the Frozen Banana
by
Joshua Millstein

Putnam & Smith Publishing Company
Cover Design by: Amit Millstein

Distributed by:
Putnam & Smith Publishing Company
15915 Ventura Boulevard, Suite 101
Encino, California 91436
www.putnamandsmithpublishing.com

Library of Congress Number: 2025948917

ISBN: 978-1-939986-64-1

Printed in the USA

Contents

Chapter 1

Preliminaries

When bananas are green, the taste is tangy and a little powdery. Then when they ripen, turning yellow with small brown spots, they get sweeter and the 'banana' flavors get stronger. When overripe, mostly brown and black, the 'banana' flavors fade and *off* flavors emerge. Bananas should be frozen when at their maximum sweetness, ripe (as in the picture below) but not overripe. Cavendish were used here but other sweet varieties would probably work fine. To avoid confusion about amount, the equivalent weight of one banana is roughly 6.5 oz. Before freezing, peel each banana, break into three pieces (helps avoid clumping), use a freezer bag, and remove excess air. Frozen bananas are easily cut with a knife, so don't worry too much about the size. For defrosting, the microwave works fine though it causes the liquids and solids to separate somewhat — both parts should be included. Actually, this process can be used as a way to generate natural banana flavoring by saving the liquid, which is flavorful and lasts a few days in the fridge. Most of these recipes will work just as well with fresh bananas. I don't mention possible substitutions, like using walnuts instead of almonds, or almond milk instead of cow's milk, but in my own kitchen, (confession coming) I almost never follow a recipe exactly as written. So feel free to make substitutions, change quantities, add and remove ingredients, use whatever happens to be around,
and follow your heart — no, your gut
(I won't be insulted).

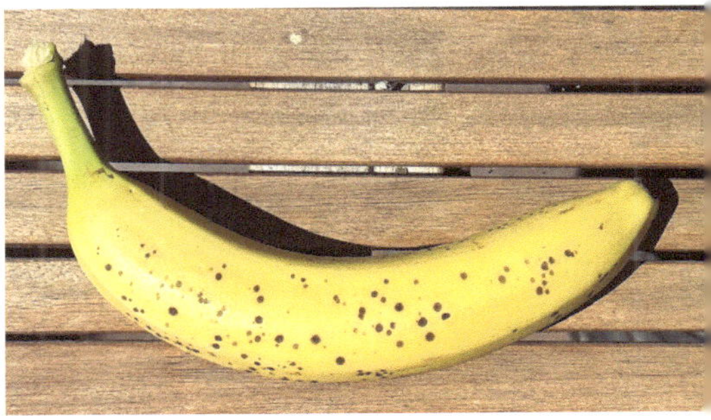

qt: quart, c: cup, T: tablespoon, t: teaspoon
min: minute, hr: hour, ": inch

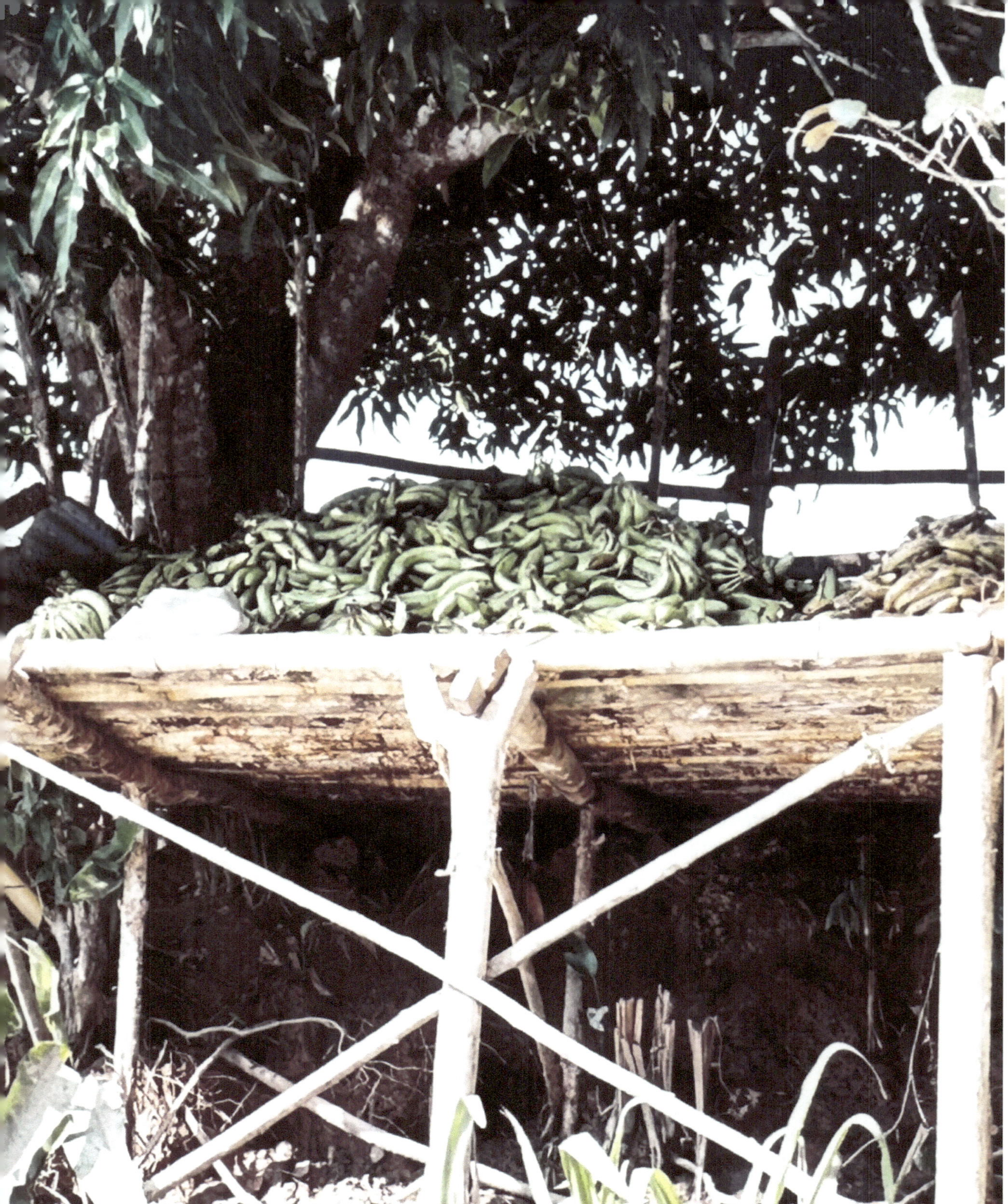

Chapter 2

Frozen Banana Inspiration

"Frozen bananas? Thats odd. Why write a book about that, even a cookbook?" (I hear you ask.) My appreciation for bananas started when I was a kid. My mom used to make "banana milk" for my brother and me by blending a banana with a glass of milk, which her mom also did for her when she and my uncle were kids. It was a delicious drink, but in my 20's I realized that if I froze the banana, it was like a real milk shake. After that, my bananas would never get overripe, because whenever I had more than I would eat during that perfectly-ripe window, I just froze them for shakes. I felt like I had to get the word out; too many people were tossing overripe bananas into the garbage without knowing they could be reveling in scrumptious shakes instead.

Another contributor was a honeymoon trip to Costa Rica with my wife in 1997. We spent a couple of weeks on the Sierpe River near a rainforest and some of the largest mangrove forests in all Latin America. On our way to the remote lodge, about 10 km north of the town of Sierpe, motoring up the river, dodging hyacinth and American and Speckled Cayman crocodiles in a small skiff, we saw something strange on one of the riverbanks. There was a meadow with a few Brahman cattle grazing and a feed pen built from wooden fencing about 10 ft square that was filled with bananas. I asked the skipper, what's going on over there with the huge crate of bananas? He explained that the bananas were supplemental food for the cows. There was a nearby banana plantation that distributed overripe or defective bananas to local livestock owners as a way to reduce food waste and environmental impacts[2].

This experience started me thinking about the role of bananas in food waste. About 5 billion bananas are thrown away by Americans each year[1]. This is partly because when bananas get ripe, there's a very short time before they get overripe, and when grouped together bananas tend to ripen all at once. My vision for this cookbook is to share dishes that I love, but also to make the case that freezing bananas is a great way to avoid tossing them. My hope is that fewer bananas will be wasted in households, and maybe, if grocery stores see a demand for frozen bananas, over-stocked ripe bananas will be frozen rather than discarded. Although there is only one recipe here that involves drying bananas (granola), it's worth pointing out that drying is another important way to reduce banana food waste[3].

I recently went back to Sierpe and took a boat up the river to look for the banana eating cows. I didn't see any, and none of the locals I talked to had ever heard of the practice. A couple of farmers who owned cattle and grew bananas in the area told me that their cows would eat bananas now and then but not as a main food source, "people eat bananas, cows eat grass." My boat guide offered a peeled banana to a calf (pg 9), but it was more interested in us than the banana.

The full page pictures in this book were all taken on that recent trip, except the one of the dock loaded with bananas for cows (pg 2), which was taken during the 1997 trip. That picture was taken at low tide — yes, the river has tides. The Sierpe River is so close to sea level that the ocean causes the river to have tides and change direction at every ebb and flow. The water flows toward the ocean during the ebb and away from it during the flow.

Chapter 3

Breakfasts

Banana Granola

15 min 5

Instructions

1. Defrost bananas
2. Mix until smooth with a fork
3. Chop almonds (a food processor works well)
4. Mix all ingredients together until the oats are well coated
5. Grease a large baking pan with olive oil and spread the oat mixture into a thin layer on top
6. Cook for 2 hours on a high rack at 250°F, stirring every 30 minutes to break large chunks
7. To make the granola more crunchy, let it sit inside the oven (turned off) overnight

Ingredients

3	frozen bananas
3 c	old fashioned rolled oats
1/2 c	orange juice
1 T	maple syrup
1 c	chopped almonds
1/2 c	raisins or dried cranberries
·	pinch of salt
·	sprinkle of cinnamon

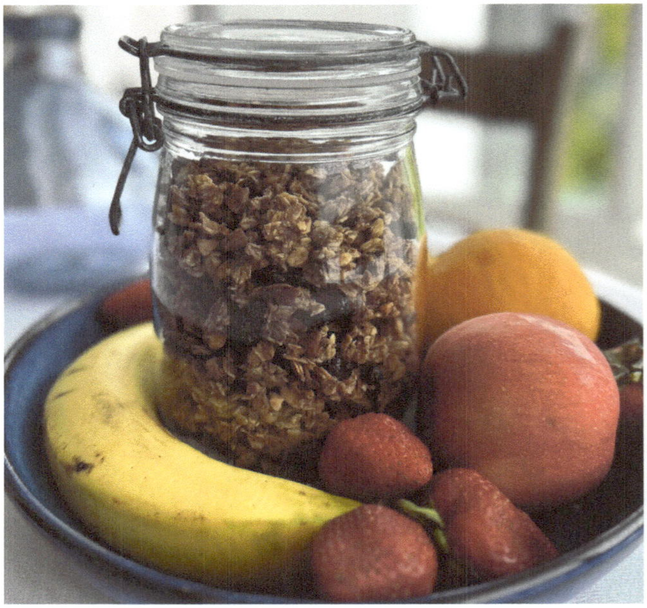

Great with shredded coconut

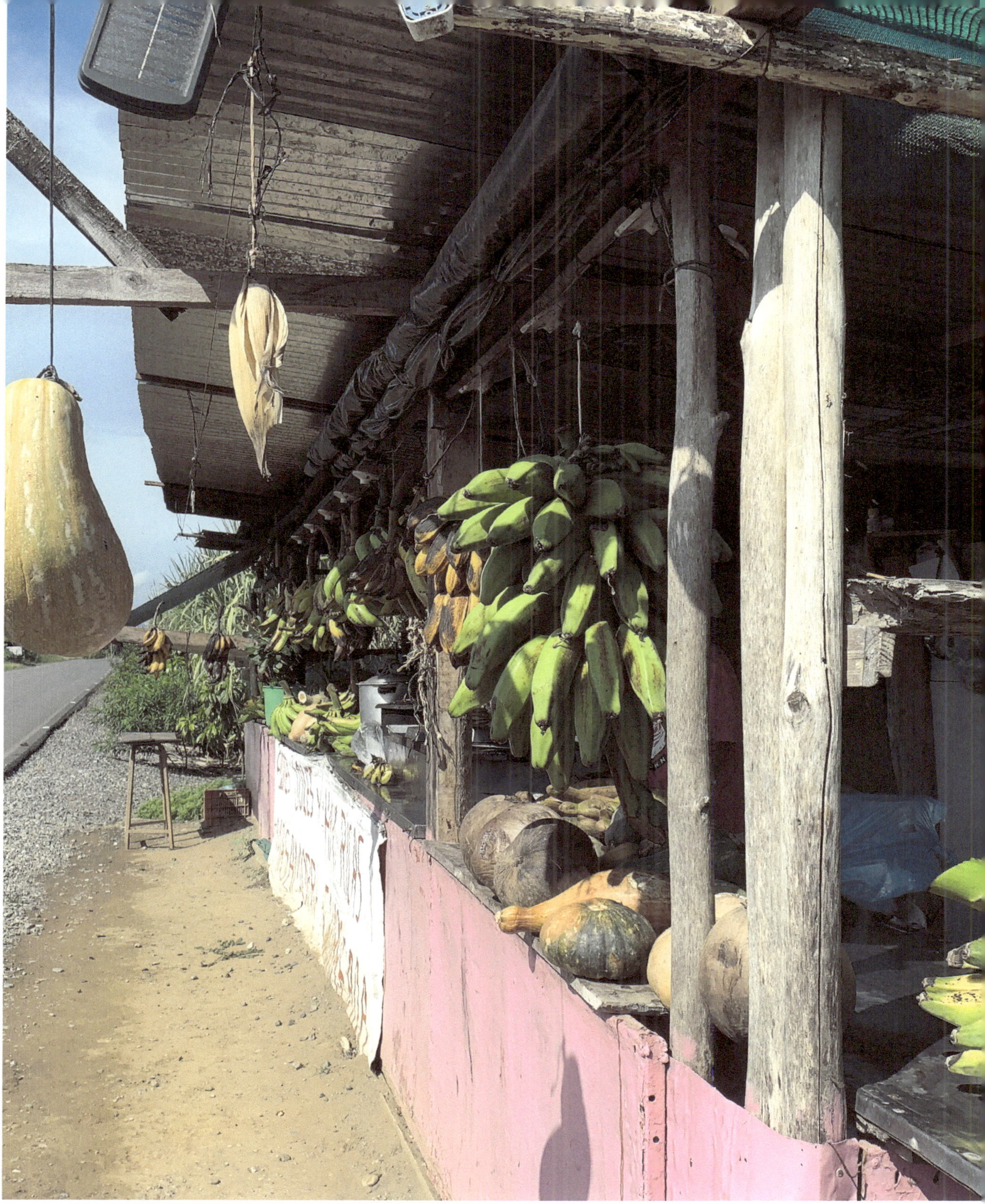

Parfait

10 min 1

Instructions

1. Place a scoop of yogurt in the bowl
2. Peel an orange, cut wedges in half, and place them around the yogurt
3. Peel and dice the mango, then layer it over the orange
4. Thinly slice the banana and distribute over the mango
5. Quarter the strawberries and scatter over the banana
6. Sprinkle granola over everything (see banana granola recipe)
7. Dribble maple syrup on top

Ingredients

1/2	frozen banana
1/2	mango
1	orange
·	strawberries
1/2 c	yogurt
1/2 c	granola
1 T	maple syrup

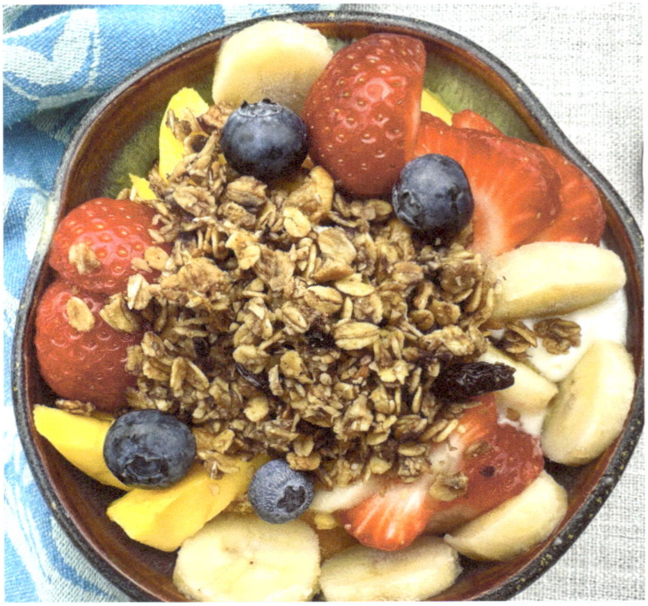

Try with nuts or a spoonful of almond butter

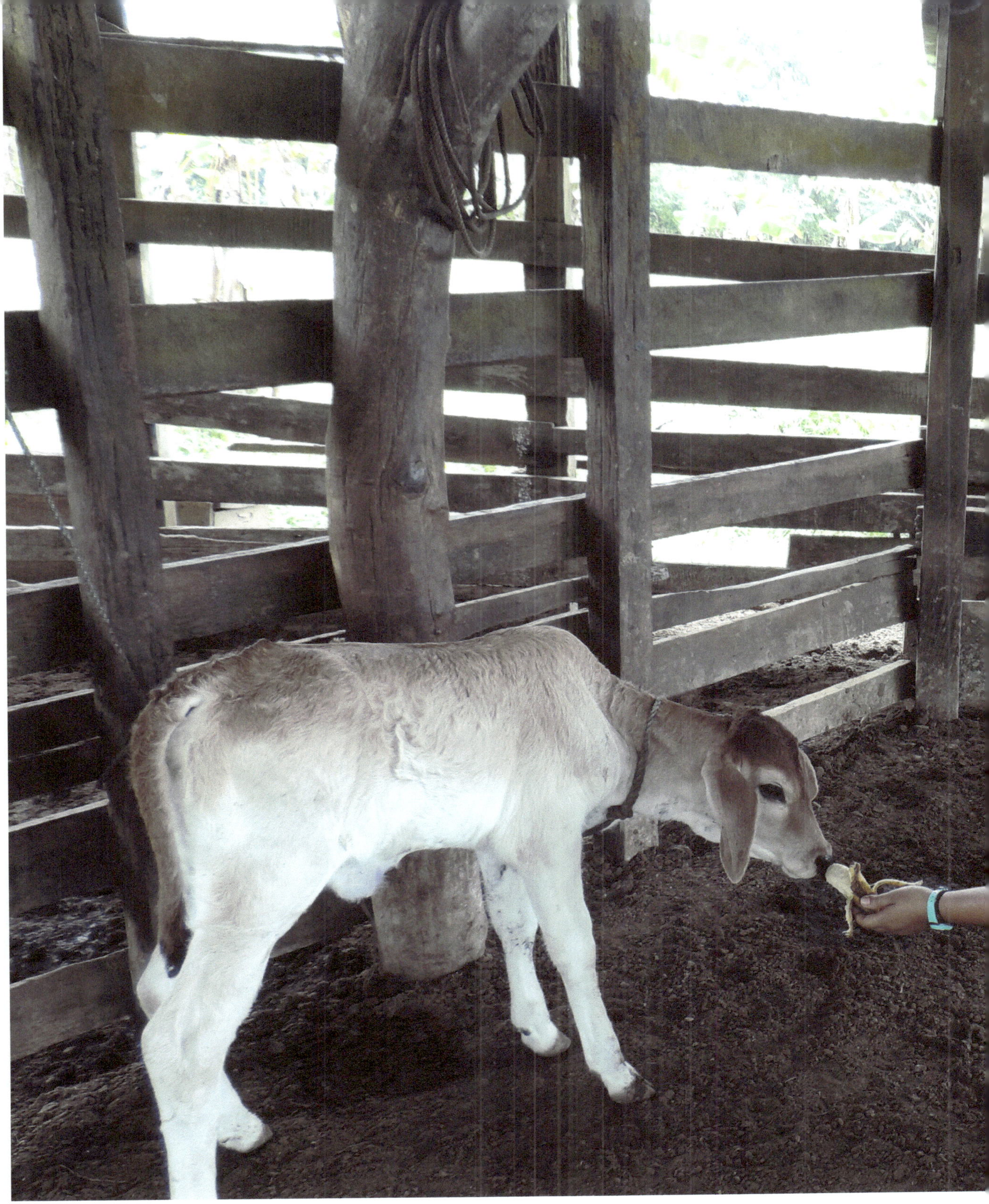

Banana French Toast

10 min 3

Instructions

1 Defrost banana

2 Mix the banana with a fork, stirring in the remaining ingredients

3 Soak the bread

4 Over medium heat, fry with high temperature oil such as canola or avocado

5 Place in warm oven until ready to serve

Ingredients

1	frozen banana
6	slices of bread
1/4 c	milk
2	eggs
1/4 t	vanilla
·	pinch of cinnamon
·	pinch of salt

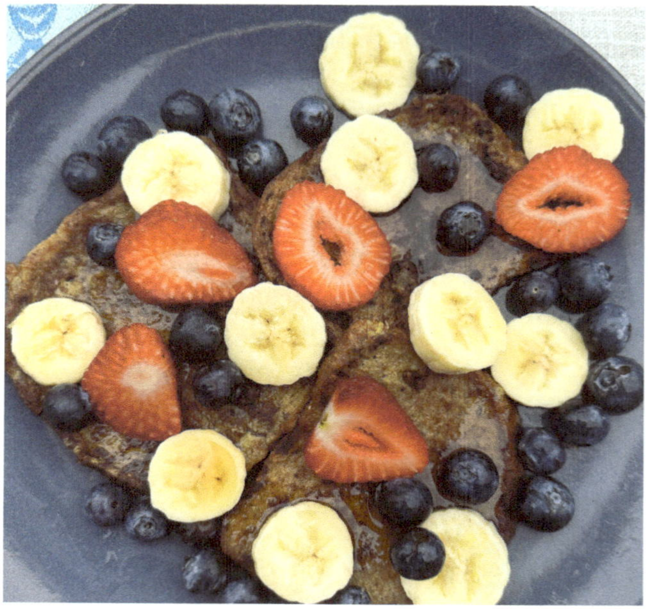

 Great with fresh fruit

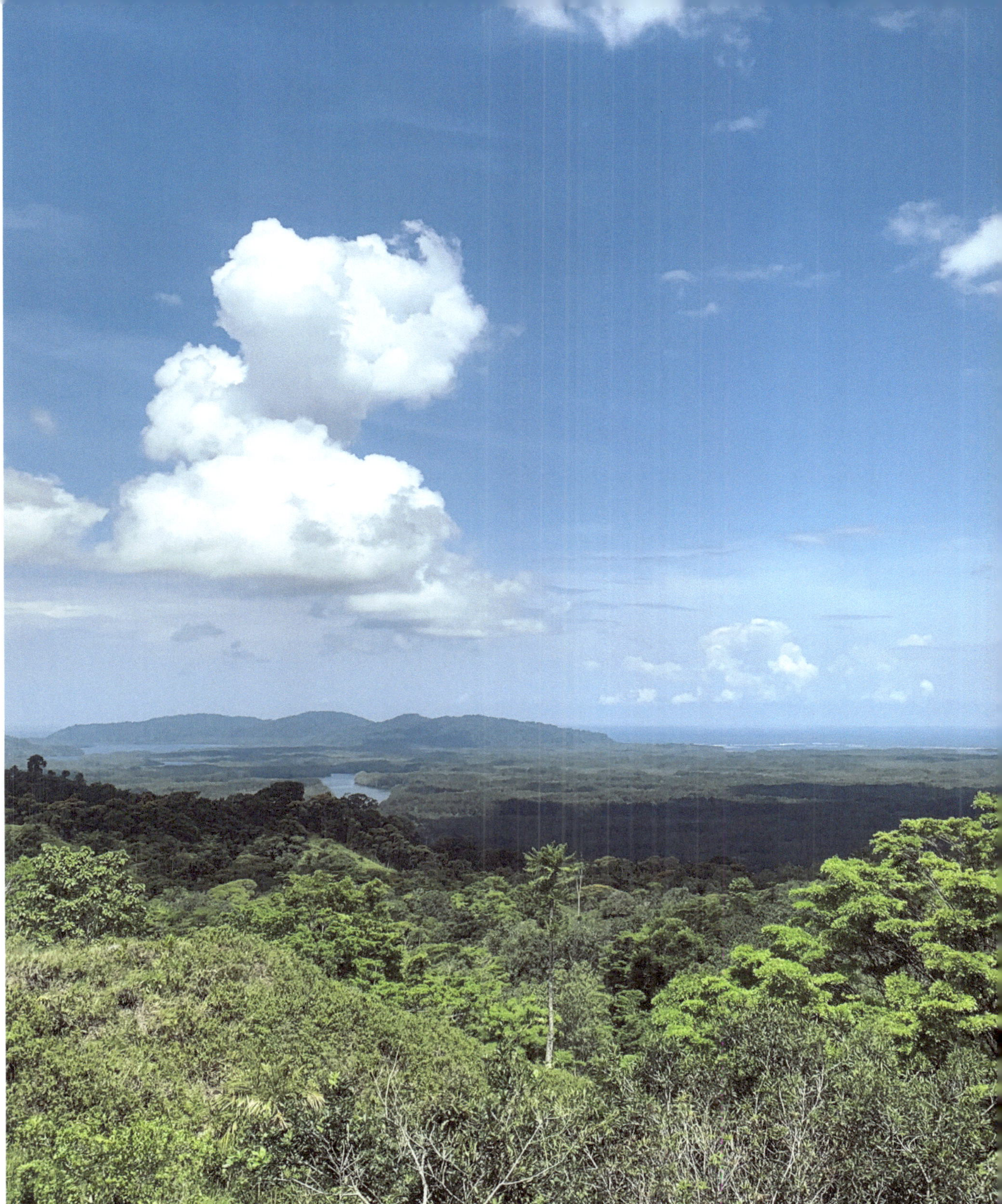

Banana Pancakes

30 min 4

Instructions

1. Defrost bananas until soft
2. Mix with a fork
3. Add the other wet ingredients
4. Mix dry ingredients in another bowl
5. Combine wet ingredients with dry and stir until smooth
6. Fry at medium to low heat with a little vegetable oil, taking care not to burn them
7. Place the finished cakes in a warm oven

Ingredients

2 1/2	frozen bananas
1/2 c	all-purpose flour
1/2 c	whole wheat flour
3/4c	milk
3	eggs
1 T	unsalted butter
1 t	baking powder
1/4 t	salt (a little less)
1/4 t	vanilla
·	pinch of cinnamon

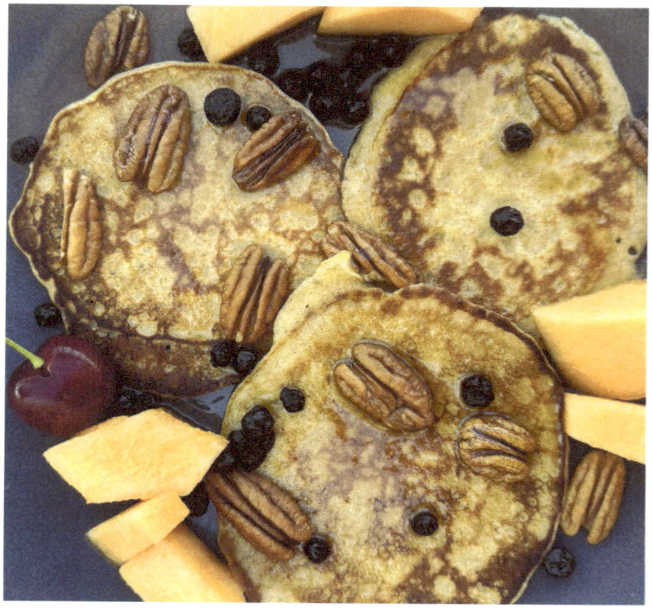

Thin pancakes cook quicker, so add water if they're too thick

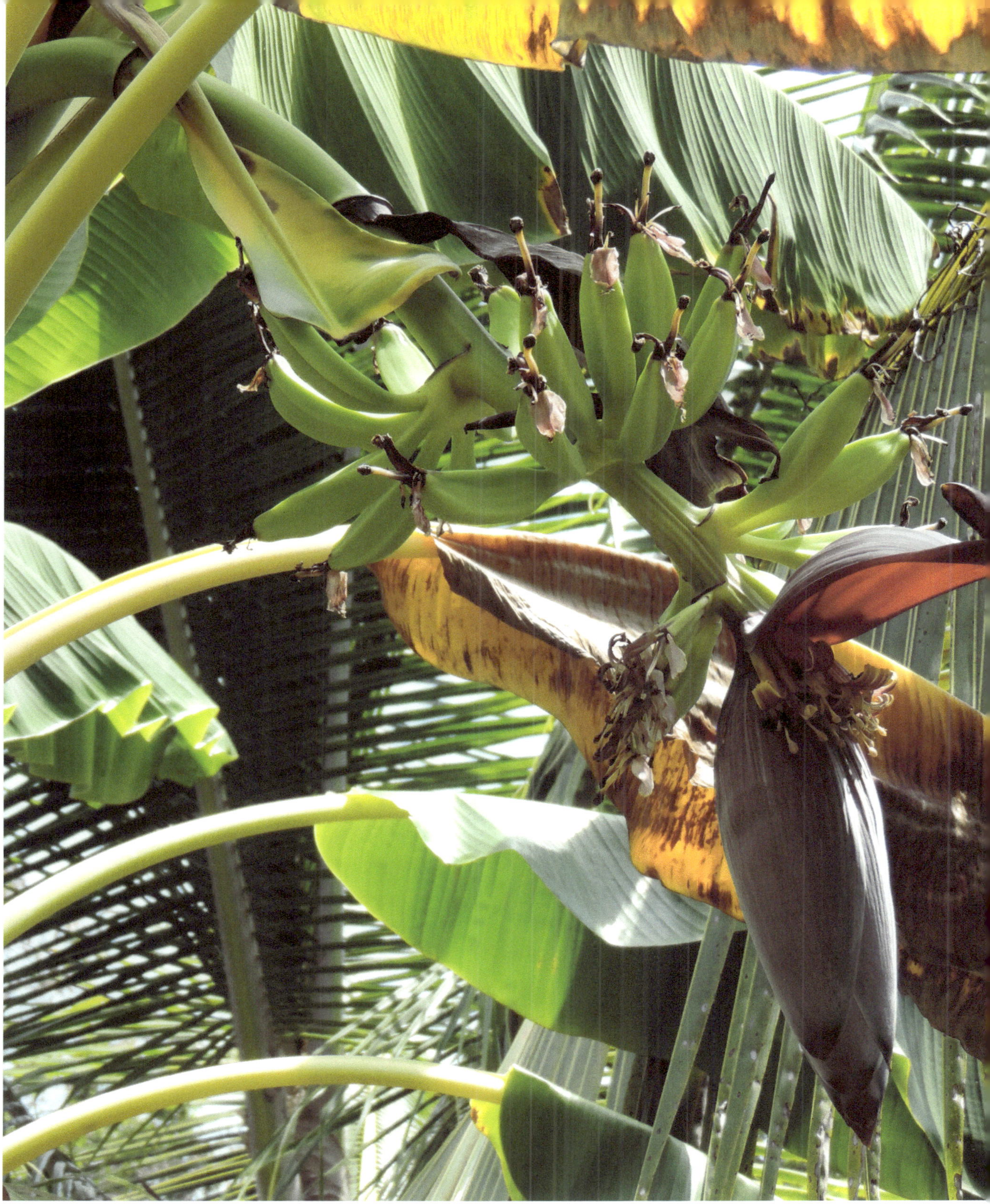

Banana Crêpes

30 min 4

Instructions

1. Defrost the banana
2. Crush with a fork
3. Mix all ingredients until smooth, using a hand mixer if needed
4. Heat a frying pan to low medium
5. Lightly coat the pan with high temperature oil and fry
6. Place the finished crêpes in a warm oven

Ingredients

1	frozen banana
1/2 c	all-purpose flour
1 c	milk
5	eggs
2T	unsalted butter
1 t	baking powder
1/4 t	salt
1/4 t	vanilla

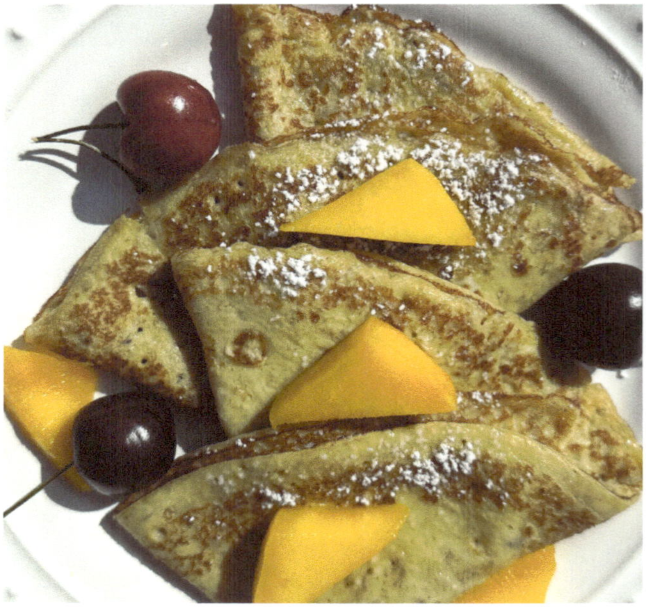

Flip carefully to avoid rips

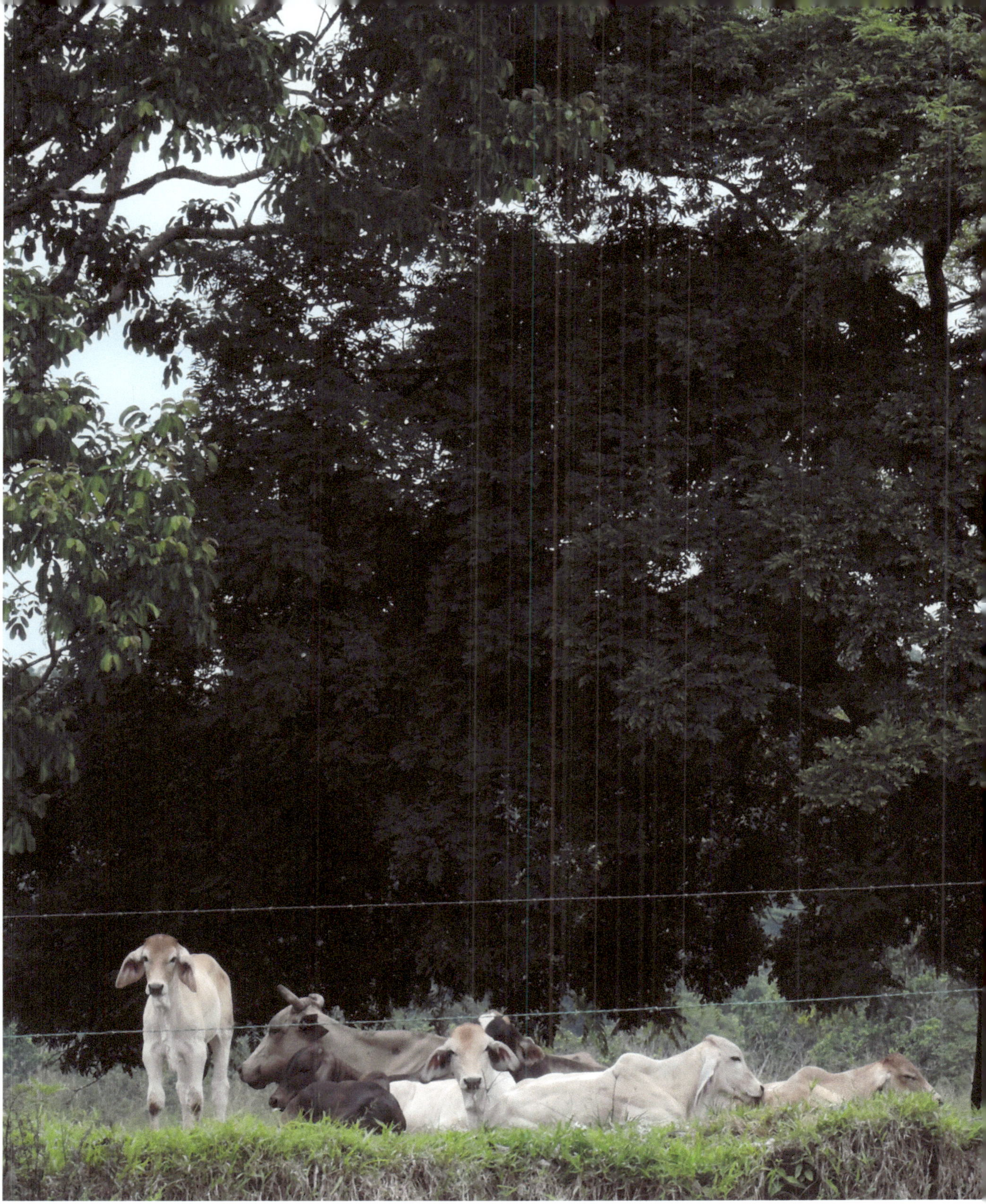

Breakfast Banana Bars

20 min 6

Instructions

1. Defrost bananas and mix until smooth
2. Coarsely chop almonds, chocolate, and rice cakes in food processor
3. Stir together all ingredients, leaving the chopped mixture until last
4. Press into an 8" x 11" baking dish, lightly coated with olive oil
5. Sprinkle some additional coconut flakes on top
6. Bake at 325 °F for 40 min in preheated oven
7. Cut into bars and let cool

Ingredients

3 1/2	frozen bananas
1 c	old fashioned rolled oats
1 c	2 rice cakes
1 c	unsweetened coconut flakes
1/4 c	maple syrup
1/4 c	orange juice
2 oz	semi-sweet chocolate
2/3 c	raw almonds
	pinch of salt

Great snack for a hike

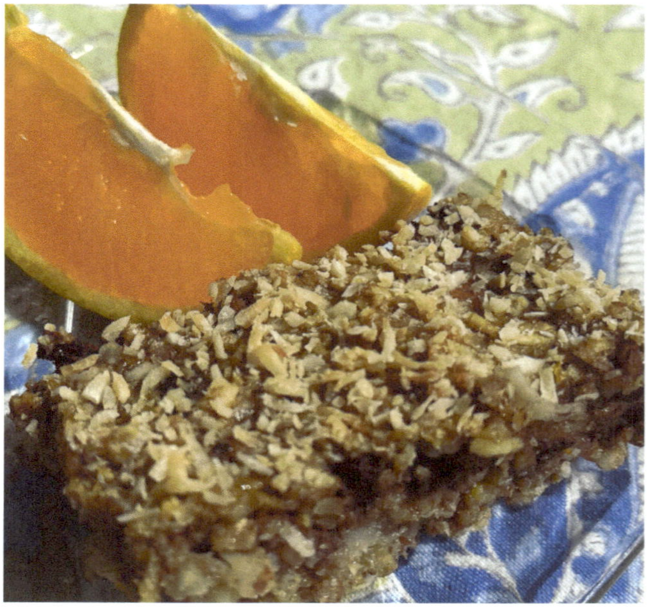

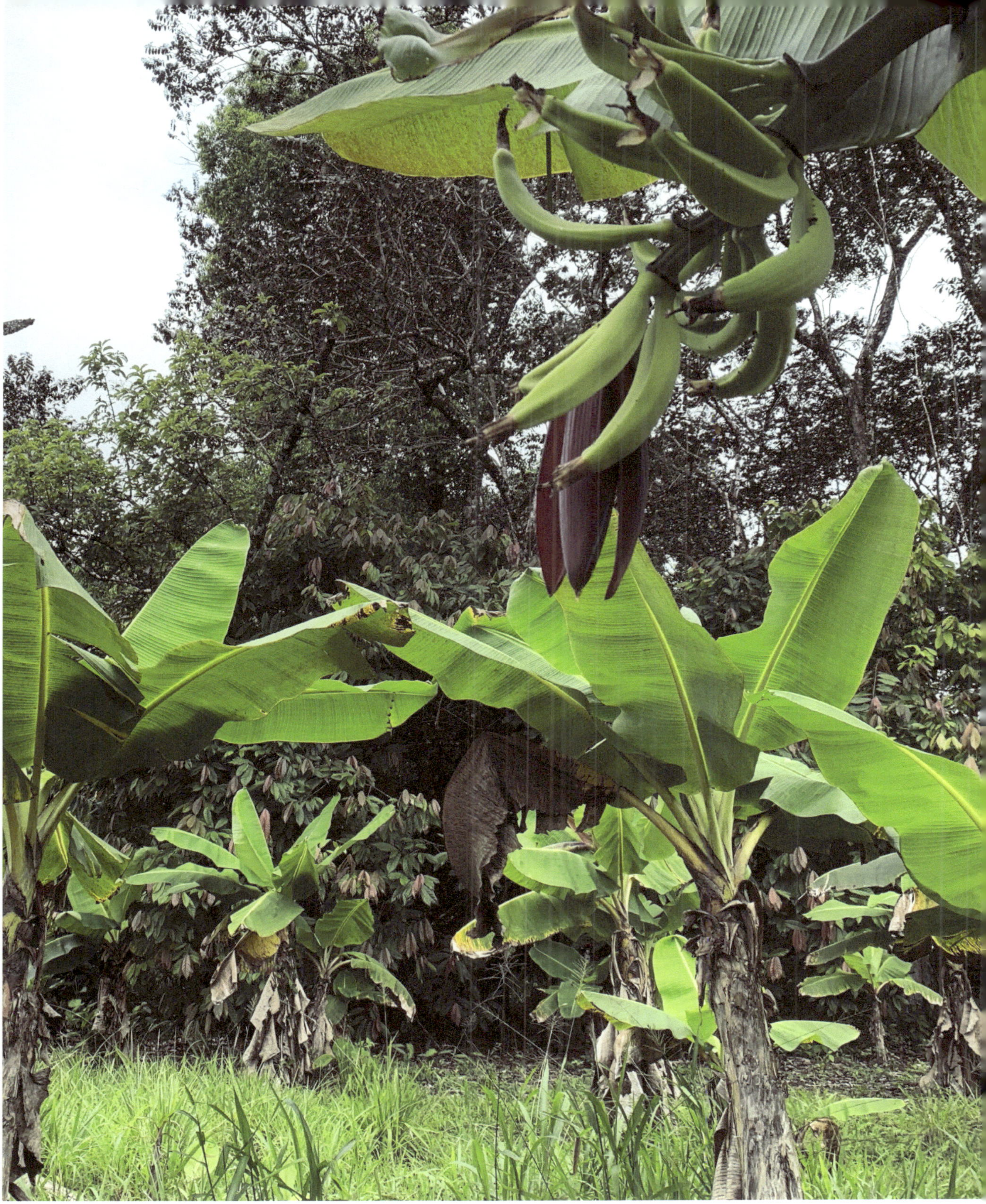

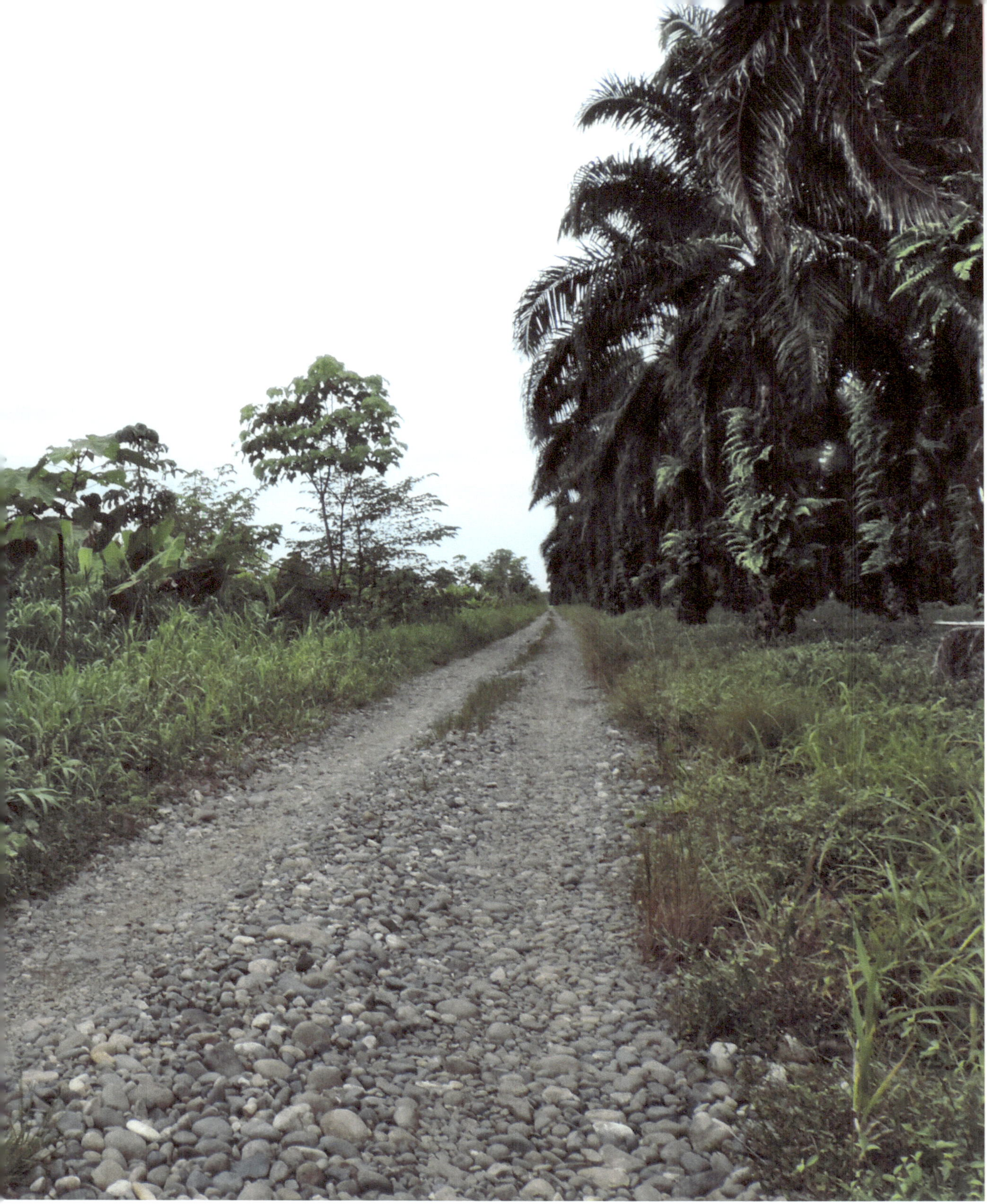

Chapter 4

Drinks (non-alcoholic)

Banana Shake

5 min   1

Instructions

1. Put all ingredients into a blender
2. Blend until smooth
3. Serve immediately

Ingredients

1	frozen banana
1 c	milk
1 T	maple syrup
1/2 t	vanilla extract
2	ice cubes

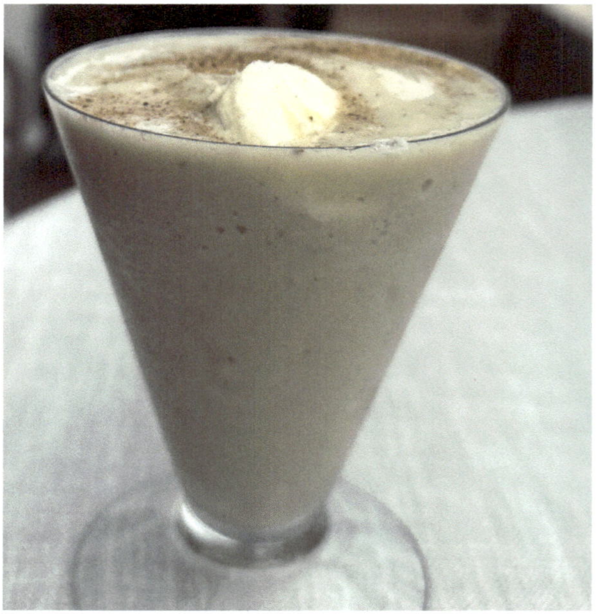

In the picture, oat-milk and nutmeg

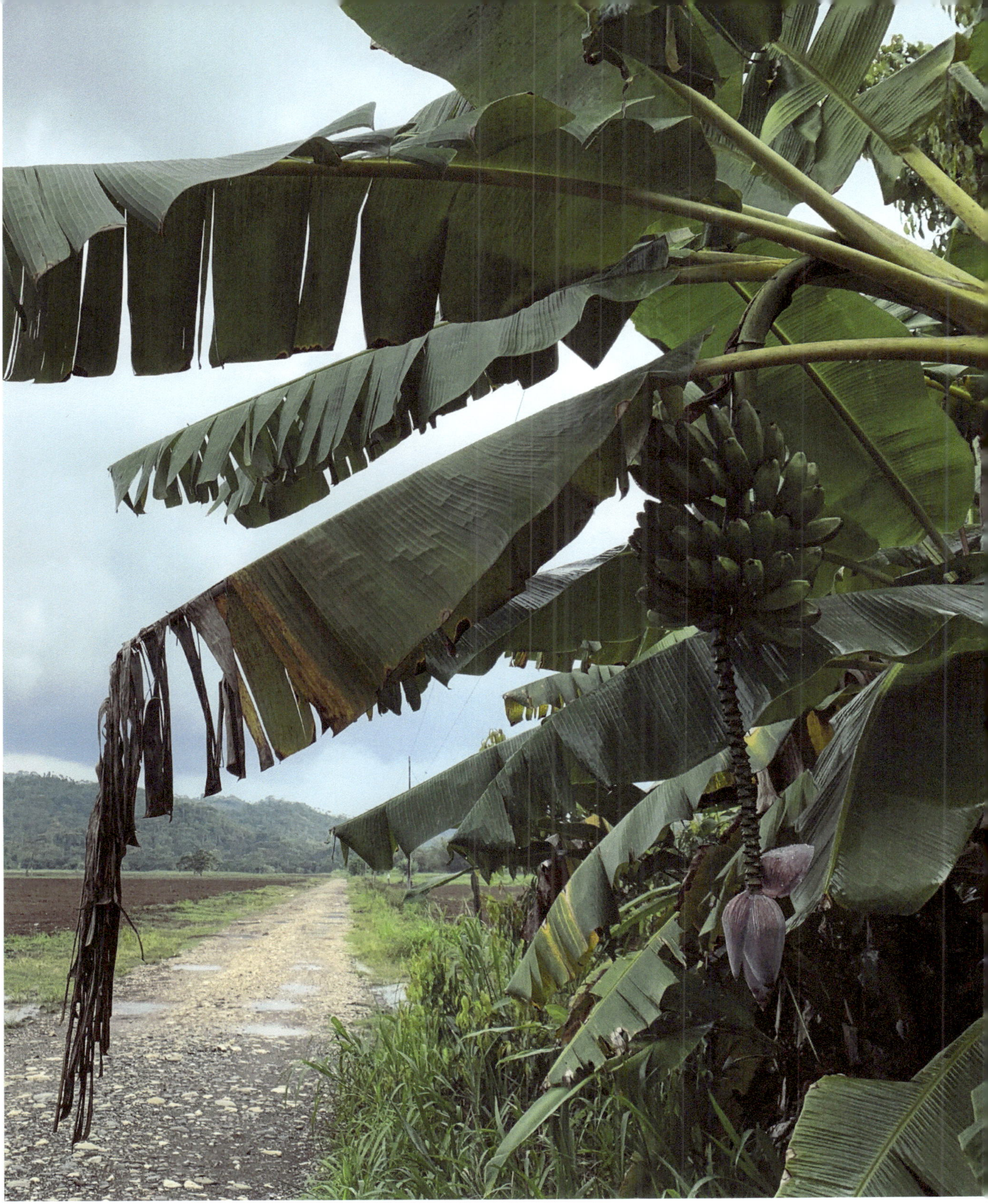

Banana Smoothy

5 min 1

Instructions

1. Put all ingredients into a blender
2. Blend until smooth
3. Serve immediately

Ingredients

1	frozen banana
1	large fresh orange (or two small ones)
1/2 c	frozen blue berries
1/2 c	frozen mango
1/2 c	water
2	ice cubes

Serve with a spoon

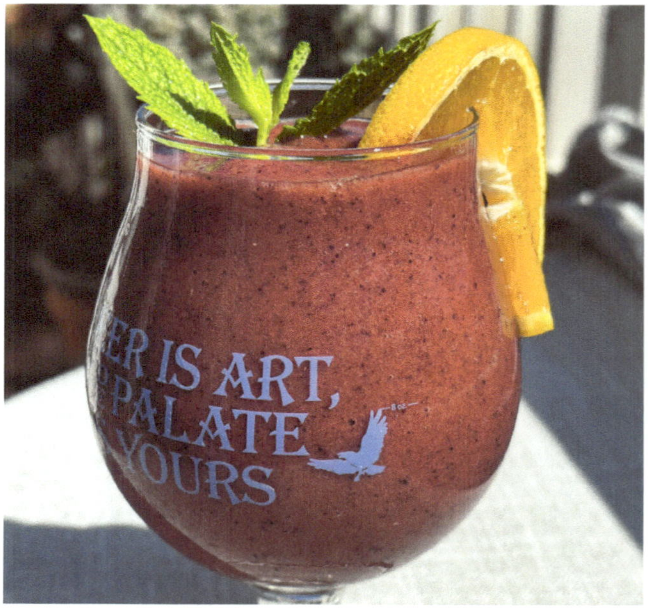

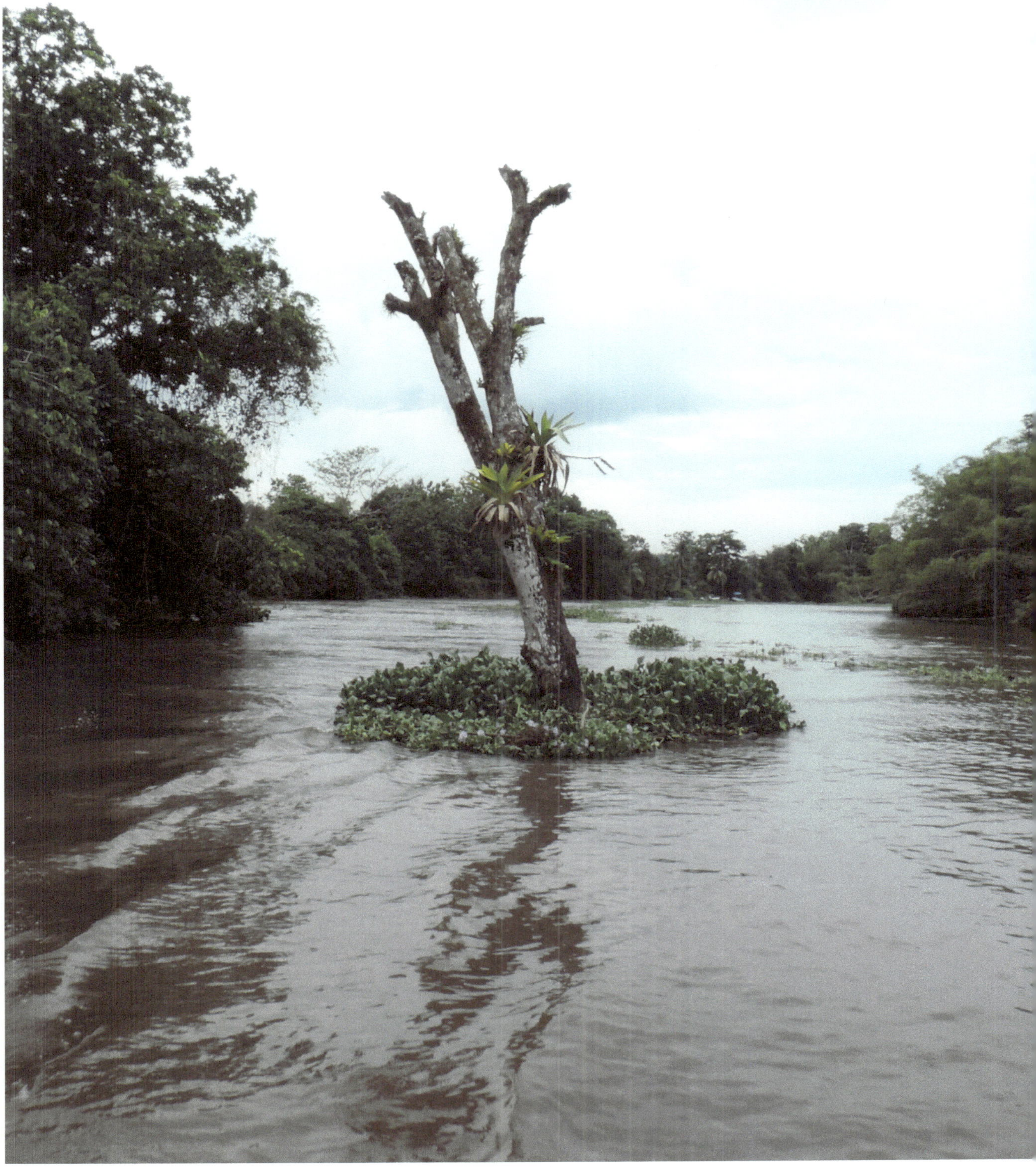

Banana Horchata

15 min 4

Instructions

1. Rinse the rice, and pour it into a blender with the cinnamon and 2 cups of very hot water
2. Thoroughly blend at the highest setting
3. Add the rest of the hot water, and soak overnight in the fridge
4. After soaking for at least 10 hrs, strain the liquid through a fine mesh sieve into the blender
5. Discard the rice pieces from the strainer
6. Add the remaining ingredients to the blender including the frozen bananas, and blend until smooth

Ingredients

2	frozen bananas
1 c	jasmine white rice
4c	very hot water, almost boiling
1/2 c	milk (oat milk works great)
1 t	vanilla extract
1 t	cinnamon
2T	maple syrup

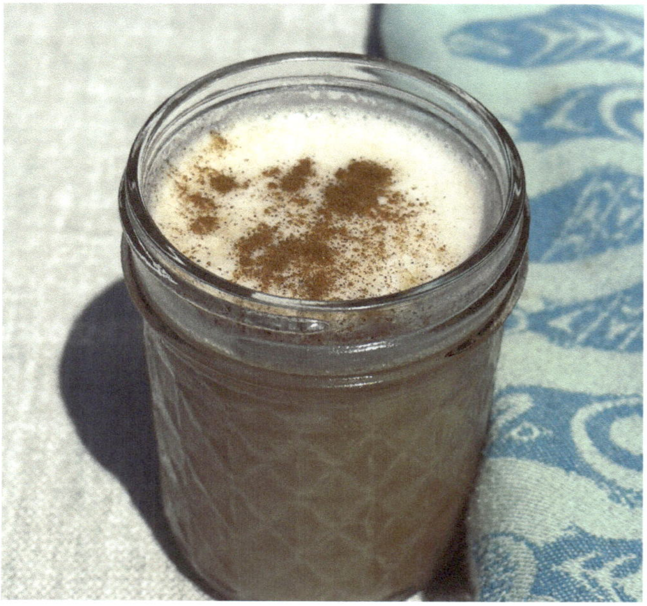

Nice over ice with a cinnamon stick

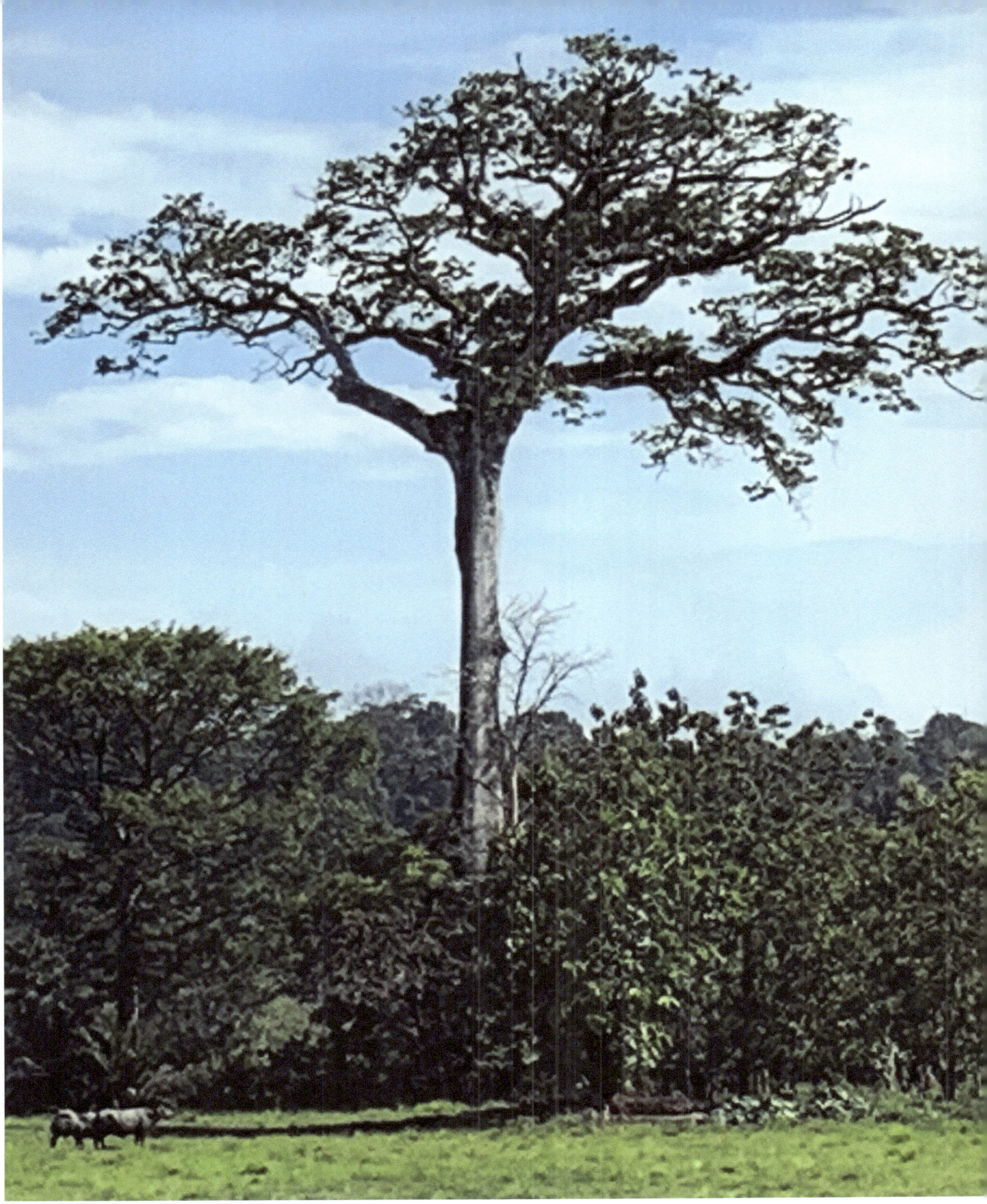

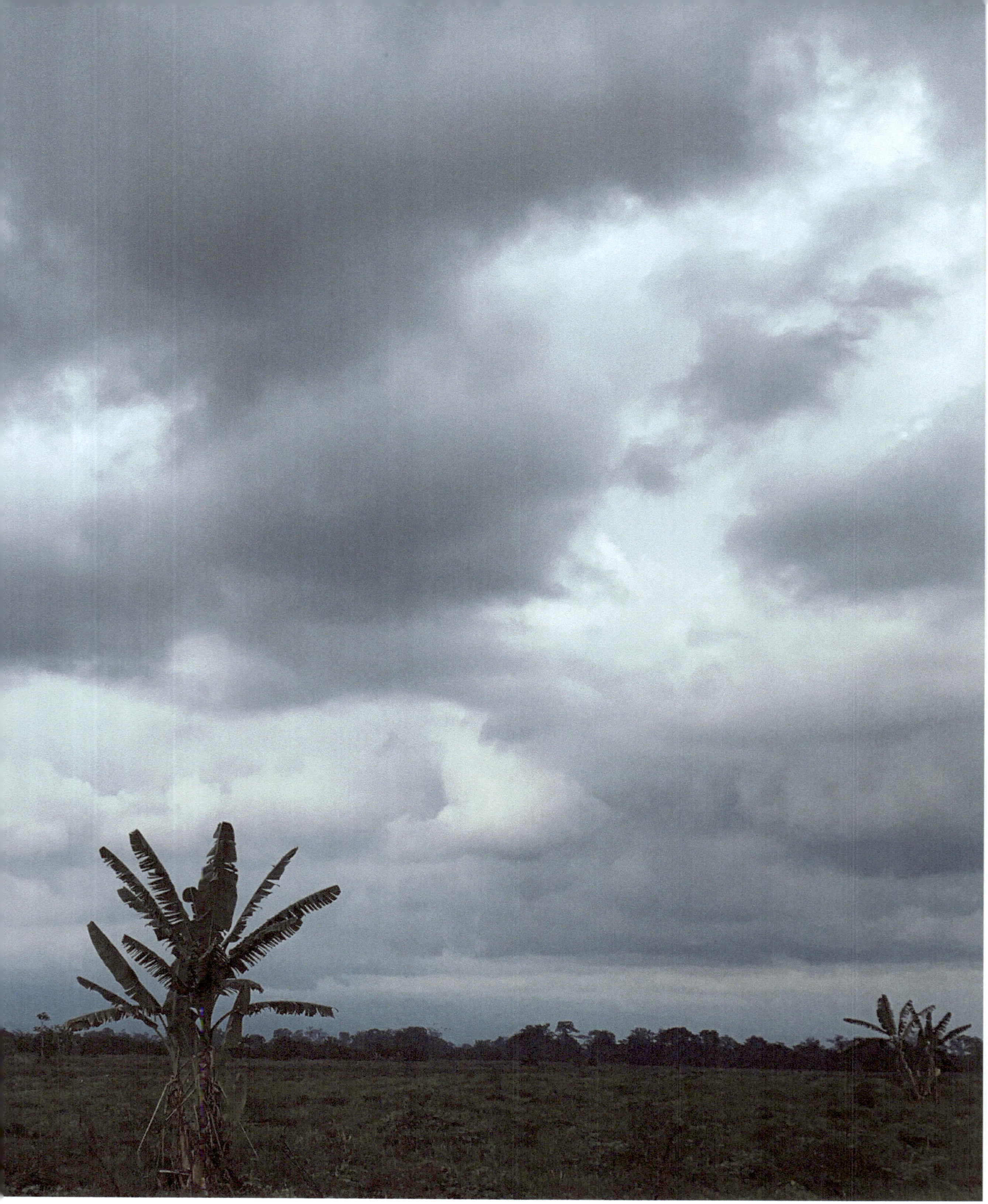

Chapter 5

Entrées

Curry Vegetables Over Banana

40 min 4

Instructions

1. Place frozen bananas on a baking sheet with parchment paper
2. Bake bananas for 30 min in an oven preheated to 400˚F
3. Sauté diced chicken pieces until golden brown then set aside
4. Cook rice according to directions and set aside
5. Sauté vegetables, diced apple, and cranberries with olive oil in large pan
6. Once onions begin to get translucent, add chicken, soup stock, sour cream, and spices
7. Simmer for another 5 min
8. On each plate, place 2 banana pieces, rice on top, and then the curry mixture on the rice

Ingredients

3	frozen bananas
1 1/2	onions
1 1/2 c	celery
1 c	basmati rice
1 1/2 lbs	chicken
1/2 c	sour cream
1/2 c	soup stock
2/3 c	dried cranberries
1	large apple
5	garlic cloves
1 T	fresh ginger
2t	curry powder
1 T	olive oil
1/2 t	salt
1/4 t	black pepper
1/4 t	cayenne

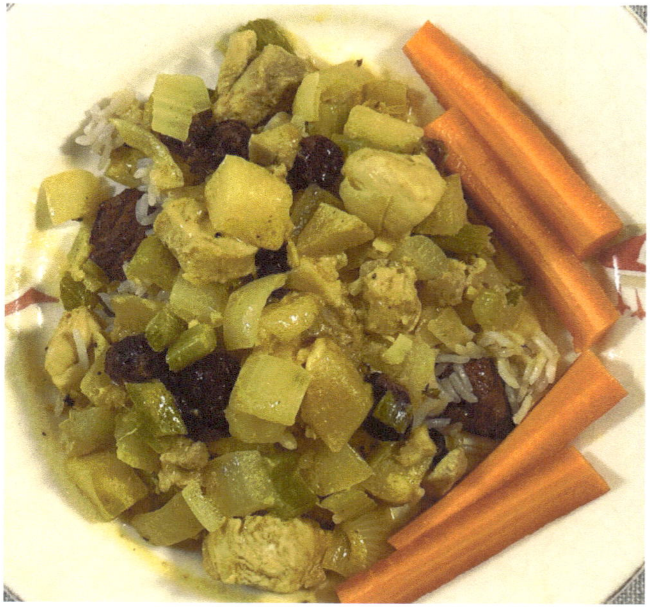

 Great with naan!

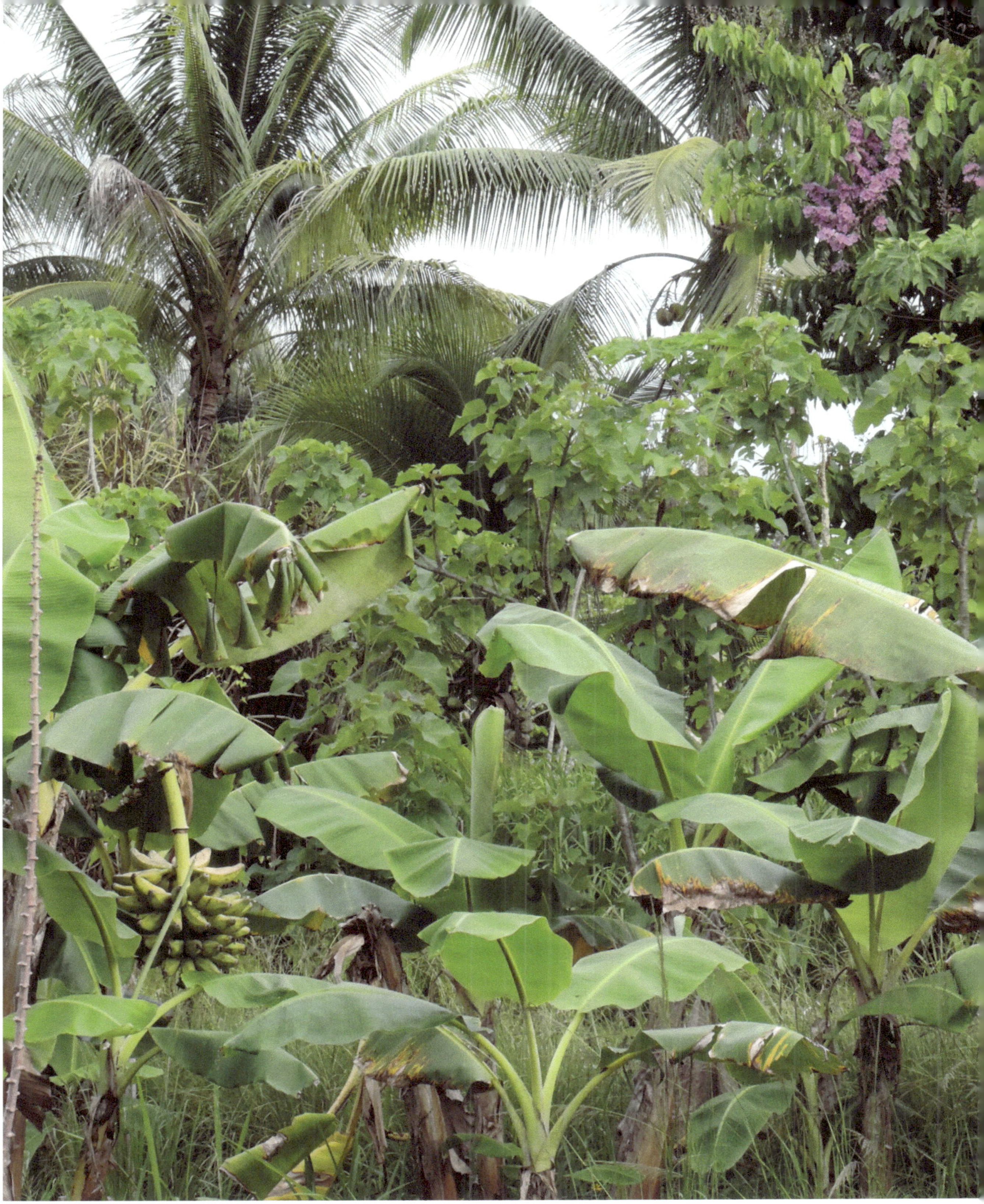

Cappelini and Banana Marbles

40 min 6

Instructions

1. Microwave bananas for 2 1/2 min
2. Collect the solid banana parts with a screen strainer
3. Mix in the remaining marbles ingredients
4. Roll into balls the size of shooter marbles and place on a baking sheet with parchment paper
5. Bake at 350 °F for 30 min in preheated oven
6. Peel and cut garlic into very thin slices for the sauce
7. Place pan over medium heat, and add olive oil, garlic, salt, cayenne, and chopped oregano, stirring continuously
8. Once the garlic starts to brown, add the tomatoes and continue stirring
9. As the tomatoes cook they will soften. Crush them with back of a soup spoon, and continue to stir
10. When the mixture becomes a smooth sauce, its done
11. Serve over cappelini pasta

Ingredients

Marbles:

3	frozen bananas
3T	olive oil
4T	bread crumbs
·	pinch of cayenne

Sauce:

3	medium tomatoes
4T	olive oil
1 1/2 T	fresh oregano
1/4 t	salt

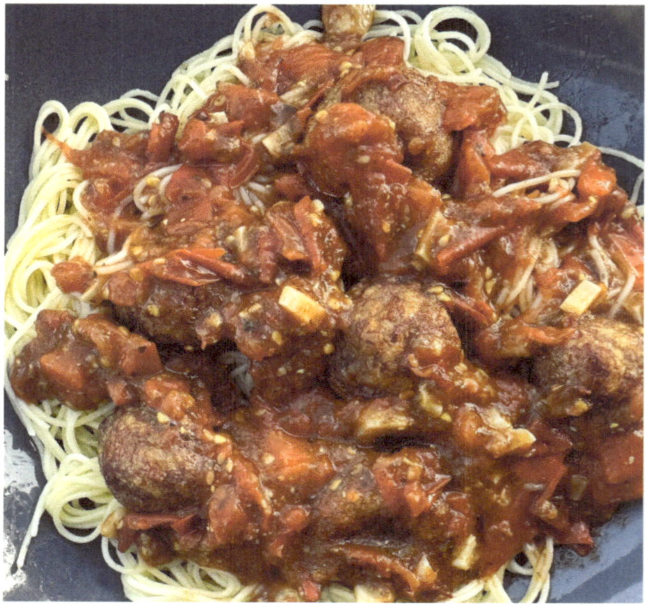

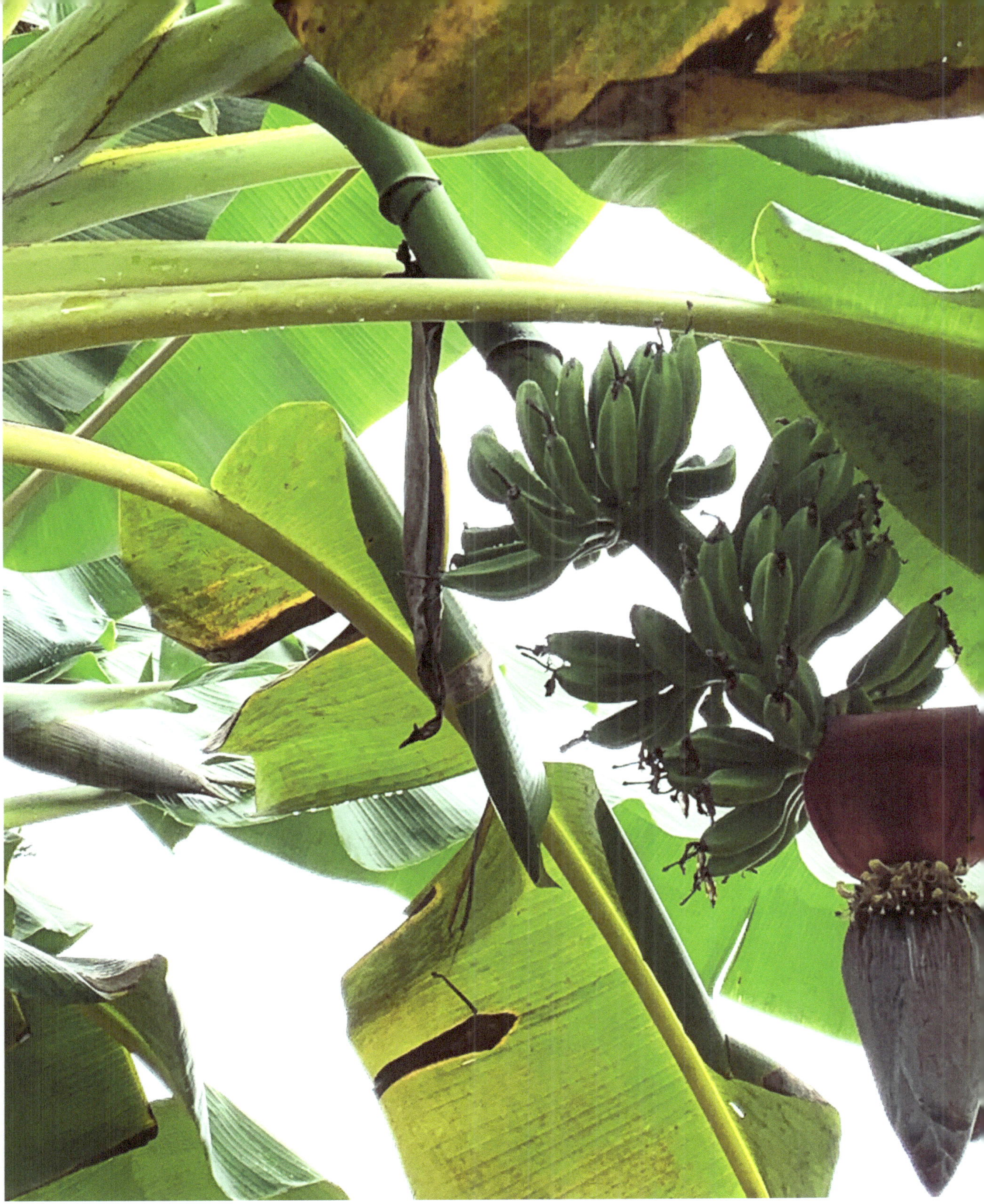

Chicken Banana Mole

40 min 6

Instructions

1. Dissolve bouillon in pot with2 c water
2. Add chicken, bay leaf, salt, oregano,1/2 onion, and 2 cloves of garlic
3. Bring to a boil and simmer for about 30 min, stirring occasionally. Remove chicken when done (save the broth)
4. In a separate pan, sauté1/2 onion with garlic and a pinch of salt
5. Once the onion is translucent, stir in defrosted banana, chocolate, remaining spices, chopped cranberries, and chopped almonds
6. Mix in 1/2 c of broth from the chicken (more if needed)
7. Add chicken and stir over low heat for5 min
8. Serve over rice

Ingredients

2	frozen bananas
2T	olive oil
1	white onion
2lbs	chicken legs
3T	dark cholocate chips
4	cloves of garlic
1	bay leaf
1	bouillon cube
1 t	chili powder
1/2 t	red pepper
1/4 t	cinnamon
1/2 t	coriander
1/2 t	oregano
1/8 t	ground cloves
1/2 t	salt
2T	cranberries
1/4 c	almonds

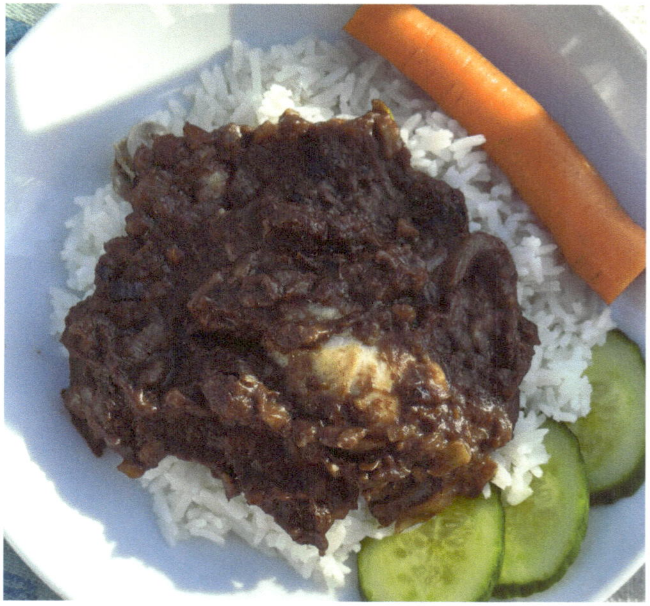

 Pairs well with margaritas

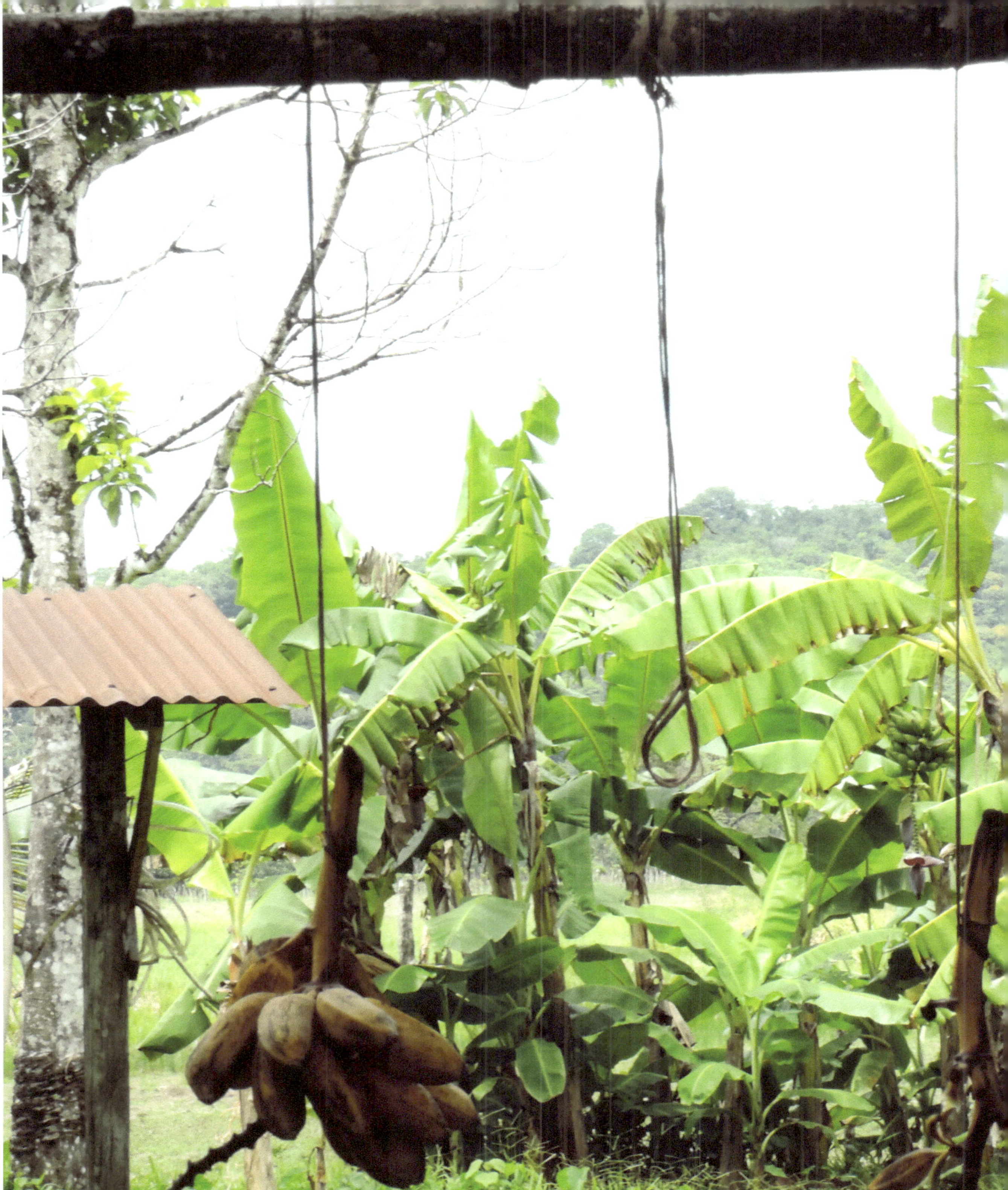

Baked Bananas and Black Bean Dip

15 min 3

Instructions

1. Lightly coat frozen bananas with olive oil, and place on a baking sheet with parchment paper
2. Bake for 35 min in preheated oven at 400°F
3. Purée the can of black beans including the water in a blender with the salt and cayenne, leaving it a little chunky
4. Chop green onions, garlic, and ginger
5. Sauté the chopped ingredients in olive oil for about 4 min over medium heat
6. Add the bean mixture and sauté for another 4 min, stirring continuously
7. Serve with sour cream

Ingredients

2	frozen bananas
1	can black beans
1/2 c	sour cream
5	green onions
4	cloves of garlic
1 T	olive oil
1 t	fresh ginger
1/4 t	cayenne pepper
1/4 t	salt

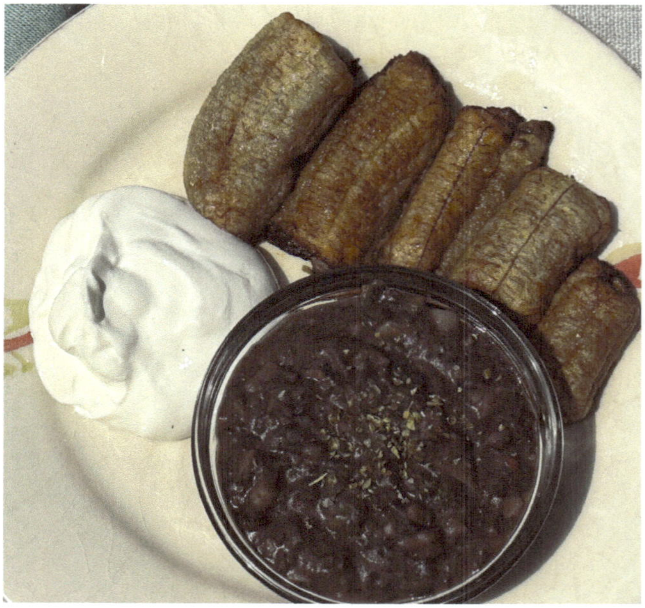

Inspired by an El Salvadoran plantain recipe - it's delicious!

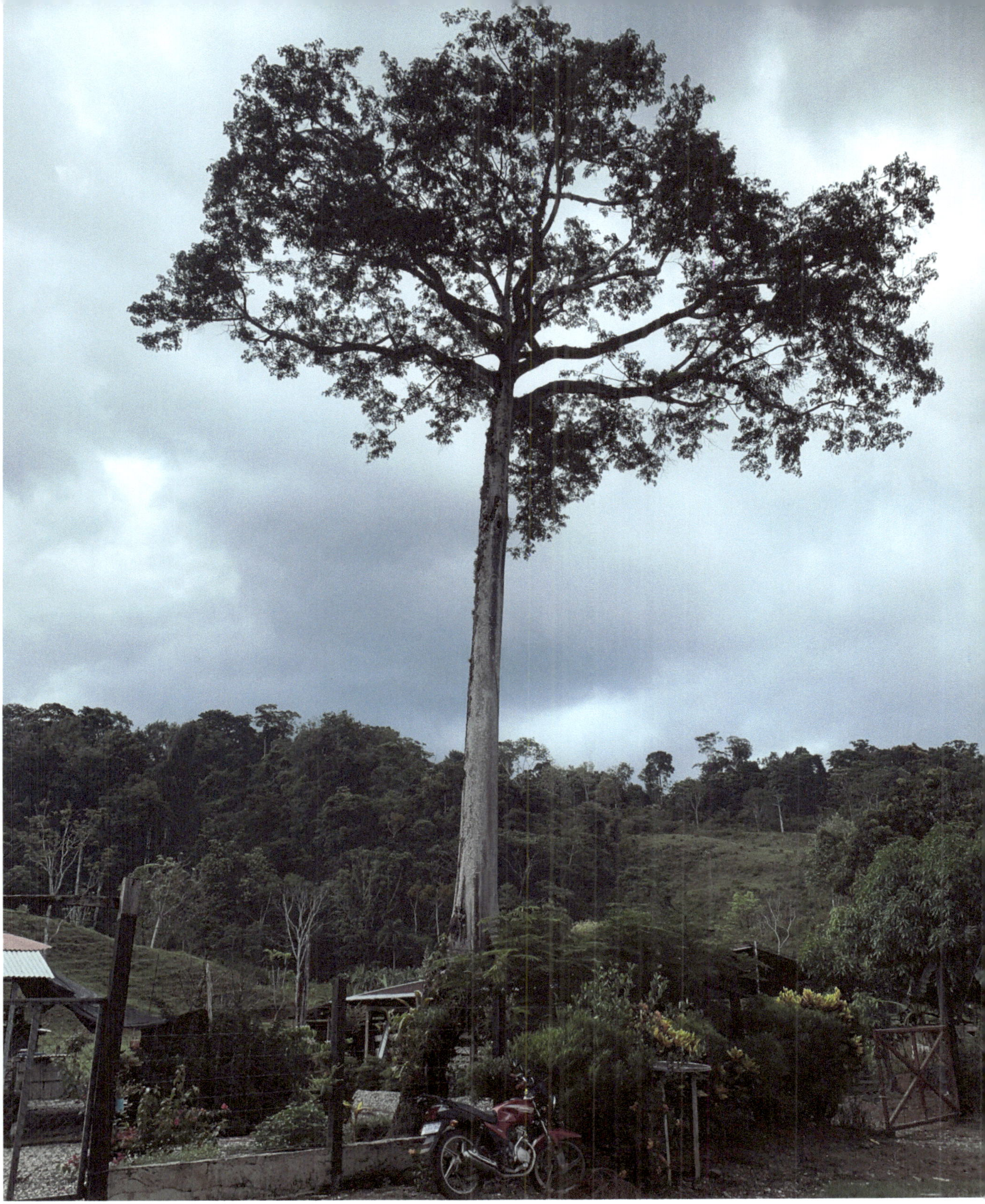

Banana Burgers

30 min 3

Instructions

1. Place frozen bananas in a microwave-safe bowl and cook in microwave for 2 1/2 min
2. Pour off any juice that has collected in the bottom of the bowl
3. Mash bananas in a fine-mesh strainer to remove more juice
4. Let sit in the strainer for 10 min
5. Mix together all ingredients
6. Shape into patties and place on a baking pan covered with parchment paper
7. Bake at 350 °F for 18 min but flip after 9 min
8. Remove the parchment paper and broil for 3 min on each side

Ingredients

3	frozen bananas
1	egg
1/3 c	chopped almonds
5T	old fashion oats
3T	bread crumbs
·	pinch of salt
·	cayenne pepper

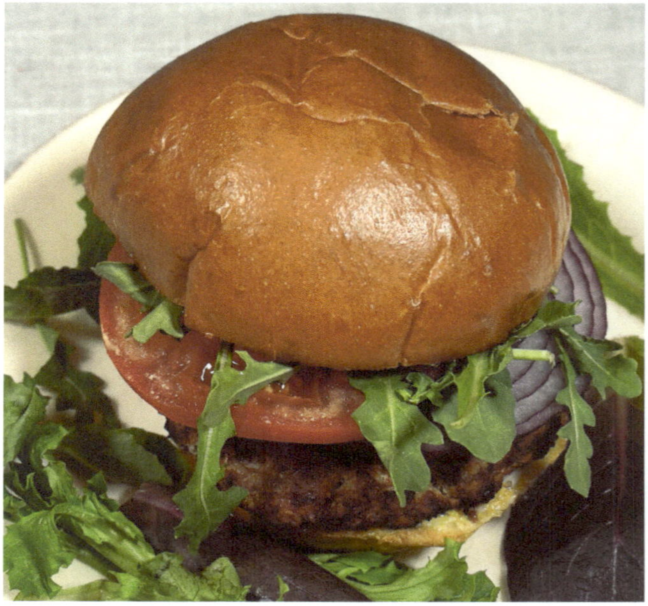

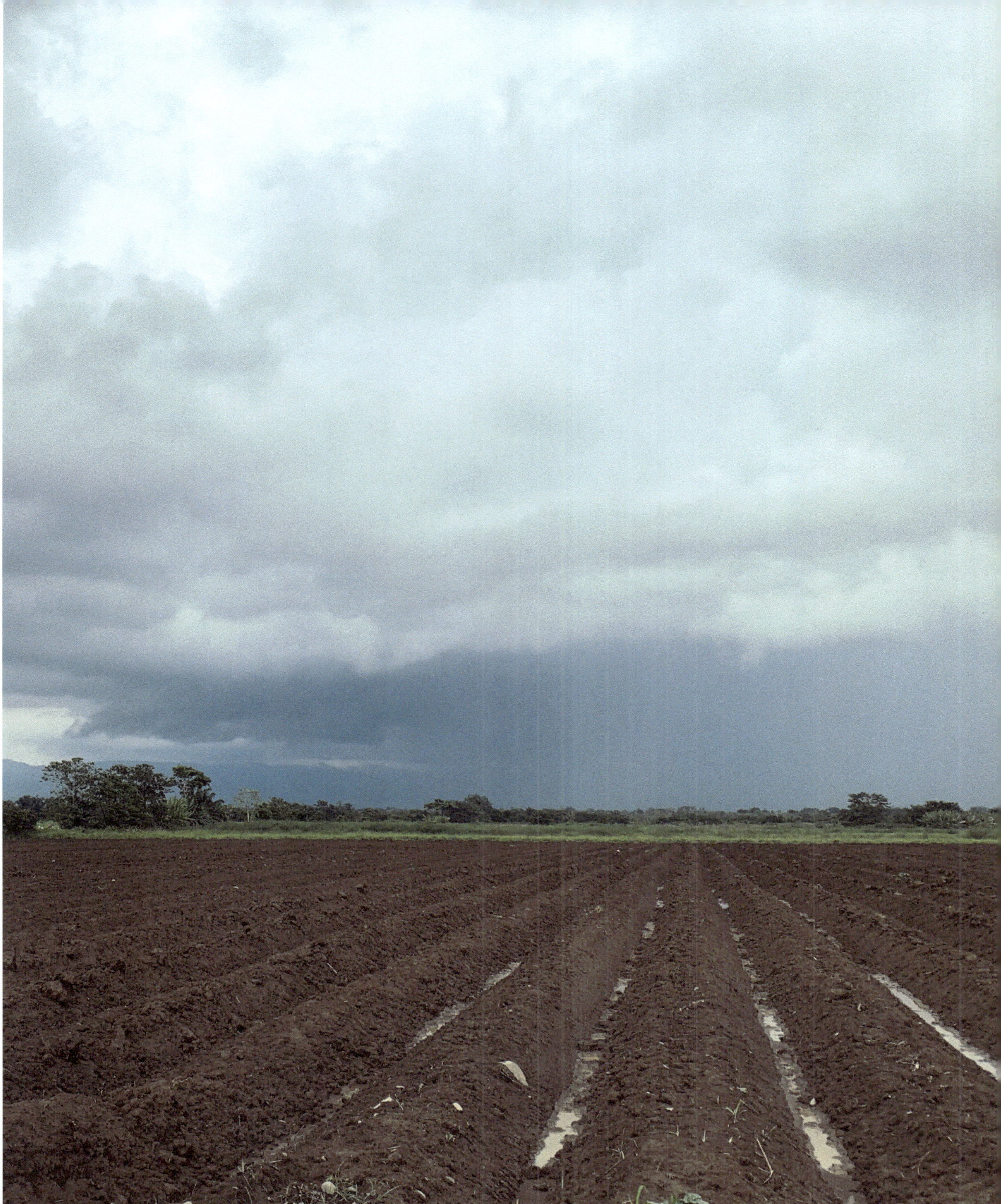

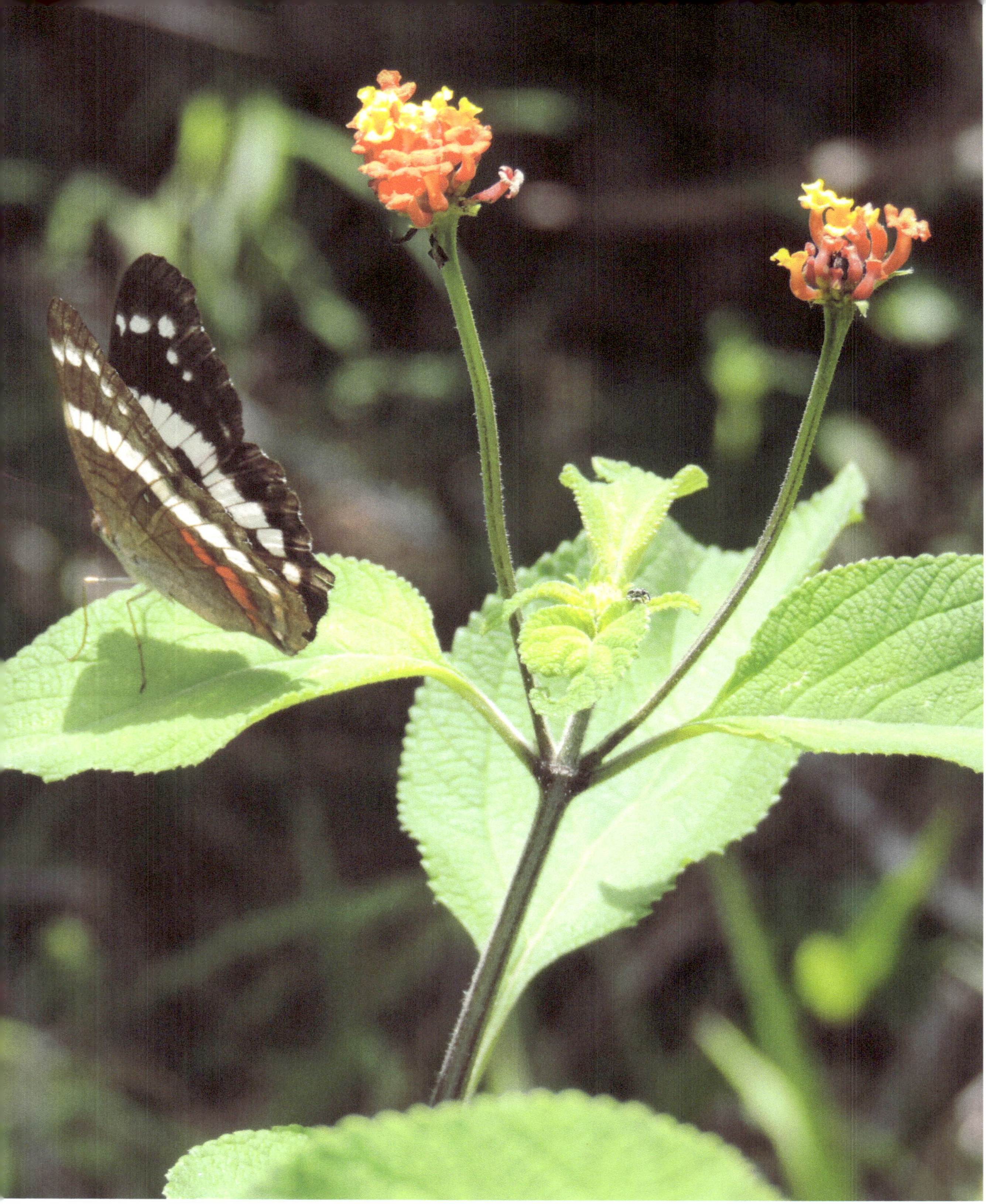

Chapter 6

Desserts

Banana Bread

20 min 6

Ingredients

5	frozen bananas
1 c	whole wheat flour
1/2 c	all-purpose flour
2	eggs
1/2 c	plain yogurt
1 c	chopped pecans
1/3 c	raw sugar
1/4 c	unsalted butter
1 t	baking soda
1/2 t	cinnamon
1/2 t	vanilla
1/4 t	salt

Instructions

1. Thaw half the bananas, leaving the rest in the freezer
2. Mix with a fork until mostly smooth
3. Mix in wet ingredients
4. Combine dry ingredients in a separate bowl
5. Stir the wet and dry mixtures together without over-mixing
6. Slice the bananas from the freezer into 1/4" rounds and delicately fold into the batter
7. Pour into 8" x 11" greased pan and bake at 350˚F in a preheated oven for 50 min. However, cover with foil after 35 min to keep the top from burning

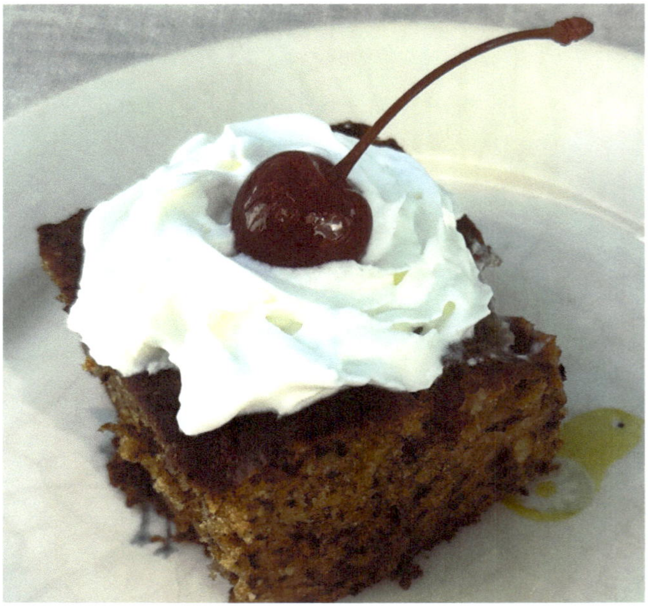

 Try a slice toasted with butter

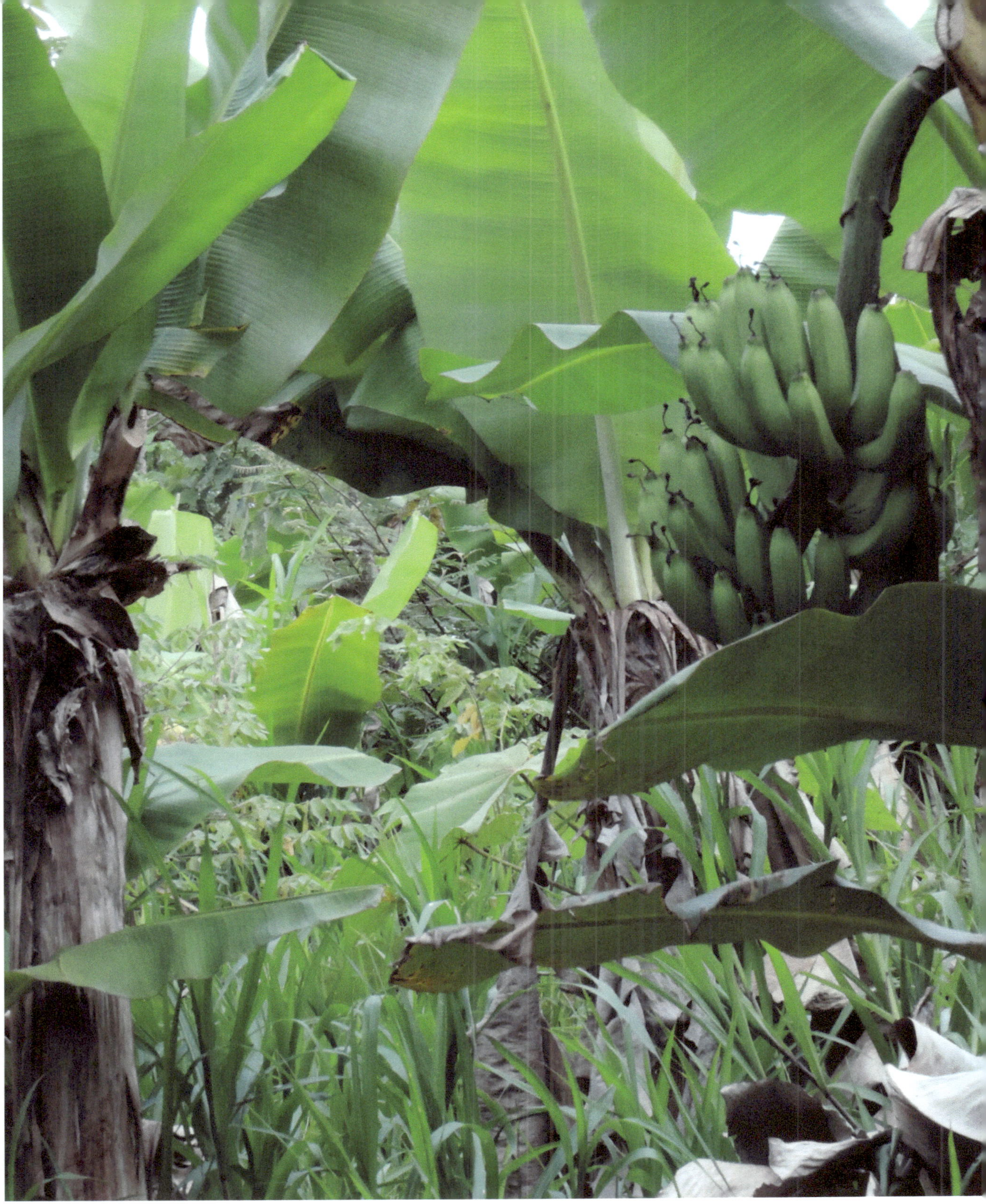

Banana Chocolate Chip Ice Cream

30 min 6

Instructions

1. Take the ice cream out of the freezer
2. While the ice cream begins to thaw, remove bananas from freezer and cut into slices
3. Blend banana slices and chocolate chips together in a food processor
4. When the ice cream has thawed for about 25 min, scoop it and the banana mixture into a large bowl using a flexible spatula
5. Stir until thoroughly mixed, but not so long that the ice cream melts completely
6. Use the spatula to put the ice cream back into its container and into another container for overflow. Place both containers in the freezer
7. Let harden for an hour or two before serving

Ingredients

3	frozen bananas
1 qt	vanilla ice cream
1/3 c	semi-sweet chocolate chips

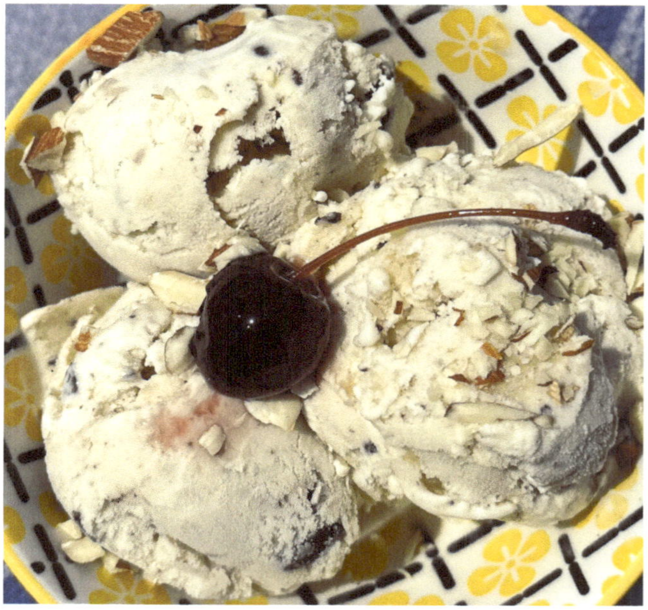

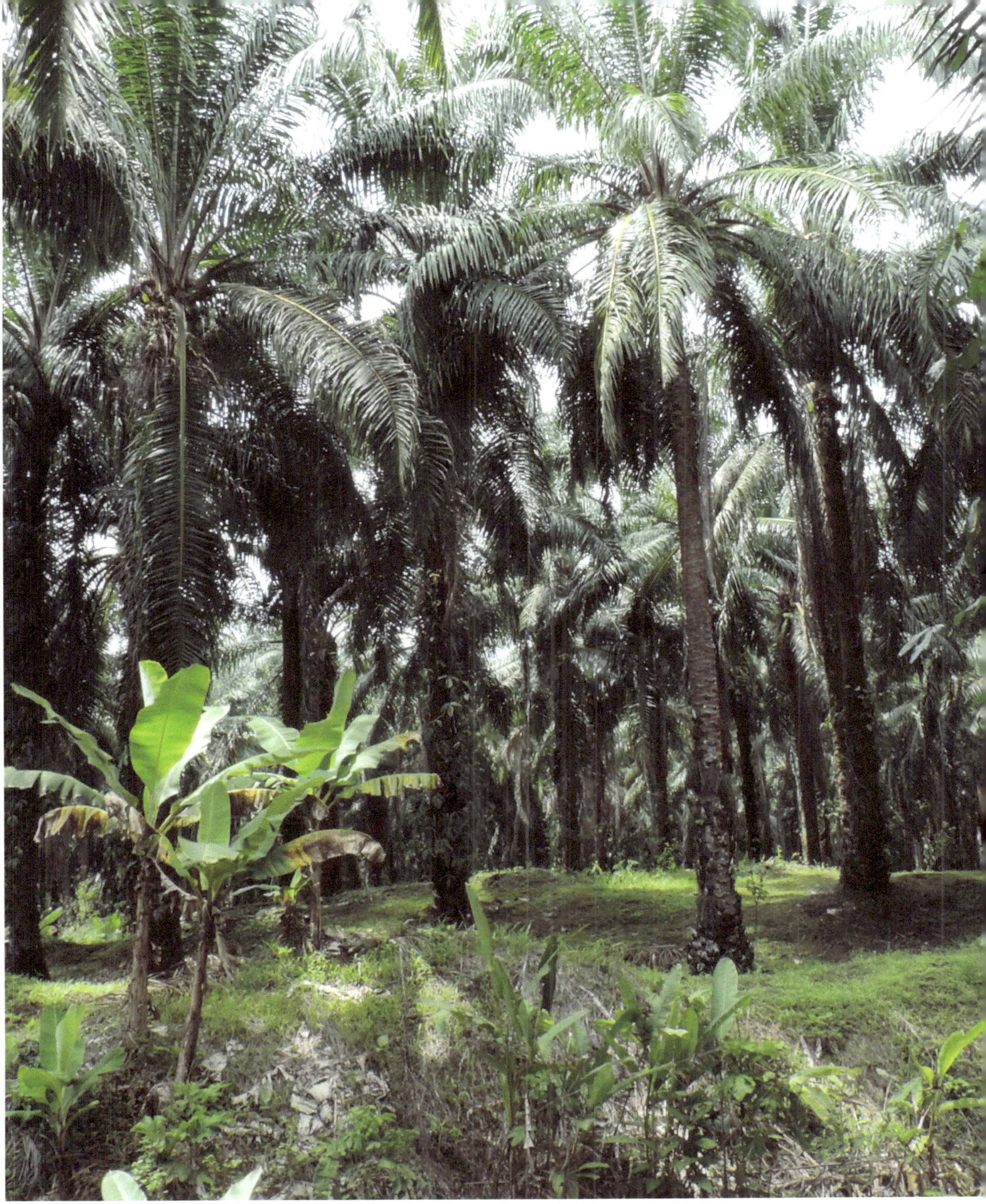

Banana Coconut Cream Pie

35 min 5

Instructions

1 Grind Grahams in processor or crush in bag

2 Mix melted butter and 2 T sugar

3 Pack into greased 9" pie pan, and set aside

4 Separate yolks, lightly beat, and set aside

5 Mix the dry filling ingredients in a bowl

6 Bring milk to a simmer in a wide saucepan

7 Sprinkle in the dry mix while stirring

8 After about 5 min, take 1/2 cup of the thickening filling and stir it into the yolk mixture

9 Add yolk mixture to the saucepan with the filling, and stir over heat for another 2 min

10 Add vanilla and butter

11 Spread a thin layer in the pie crust

12 Layer in 1/4" slices of bananas, then the remaining filling on top, covering all the banana pieces completely

13 Cover and cool in the refrigerator for 4 hrs

14 Sprinkle coconut flakes on top before serving

Ingredients

1 3/4 c	Graham crackers
5T	unsalted butter
2T	raw sugar (crust)
3	frozen bananas
3c	milk
1/3 c	all-purpose flour
1/2 c	raw sugar (filling)
3	egg yolks
1 T	unsalted butter
1 c	coconut flakes
1 t	vanilla extract
1/4 t	salt

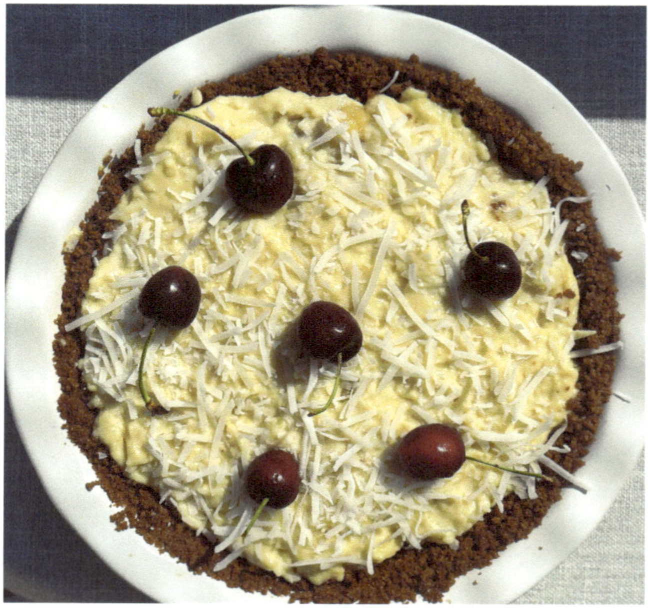

Avoid burning the filling by using low heat and stirring a lot

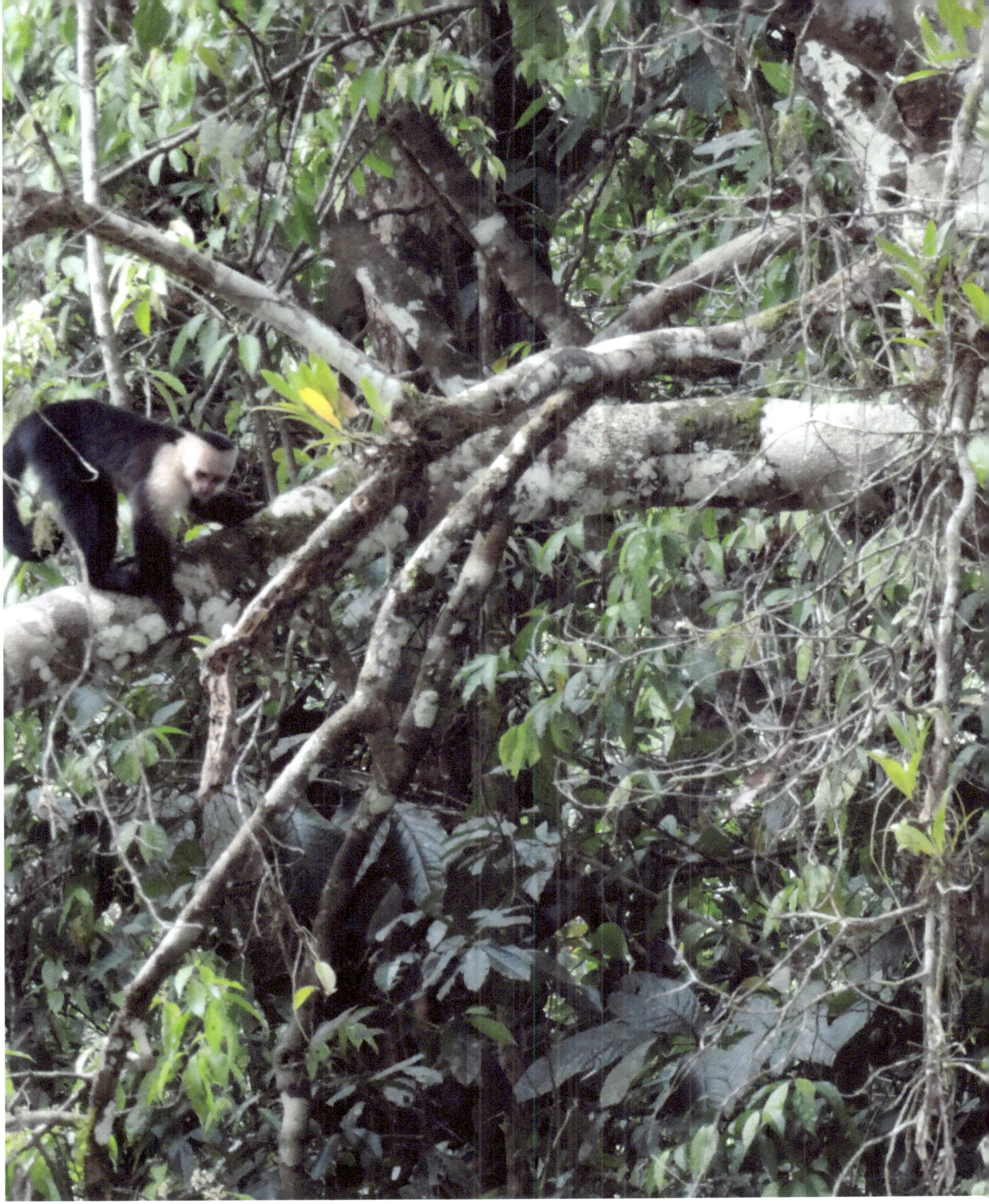

Banana Bon Bons

35 min 4

Instructions

1. Slice bananas into 1/2" rounds and place in a bowl in the freezer
2. Heat about 1" of water just shy of a simmer in a pan
3. Place a heat-tolerant bowl in the hot water
4. Break the chocolate into pieces and put them in the hot bowl along with the oil
5. Stir continuously until the chocolate is completely melted
6. Place a bowl with the chopped cashews nearby, along with parchment paper on a baking sheet
7. One-by-one, take each banana piece out of the freezer and roll it around in the chocolate using a spoon
8. Then, roll it in the cashew pieces and put it on the baking sheet
9. Once all pieces are on the sheet, place it in the freezer to cool for about 1/2 hr

Ingredients

2	frozen bananas
1 c	finely chopped roasted cashews
6oz	70-75% dark chocolate (your favorite bar)
1 T	avocado oil (canola will work fine)

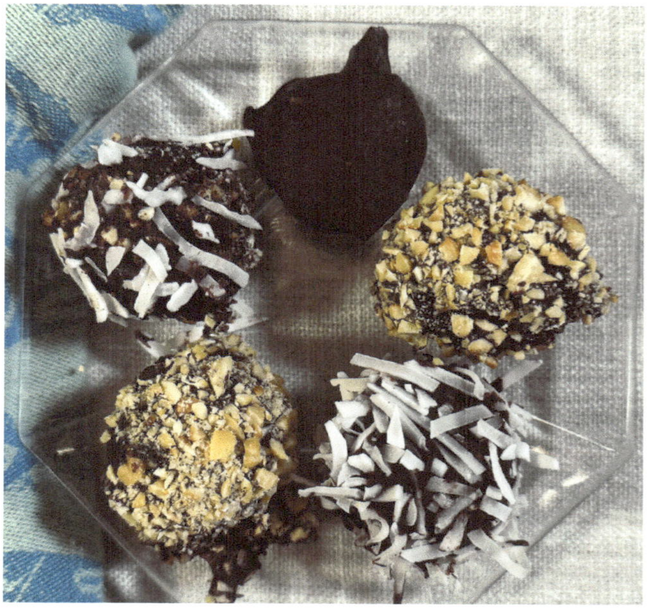

Cold bananas and hot chocolate are the keys to success

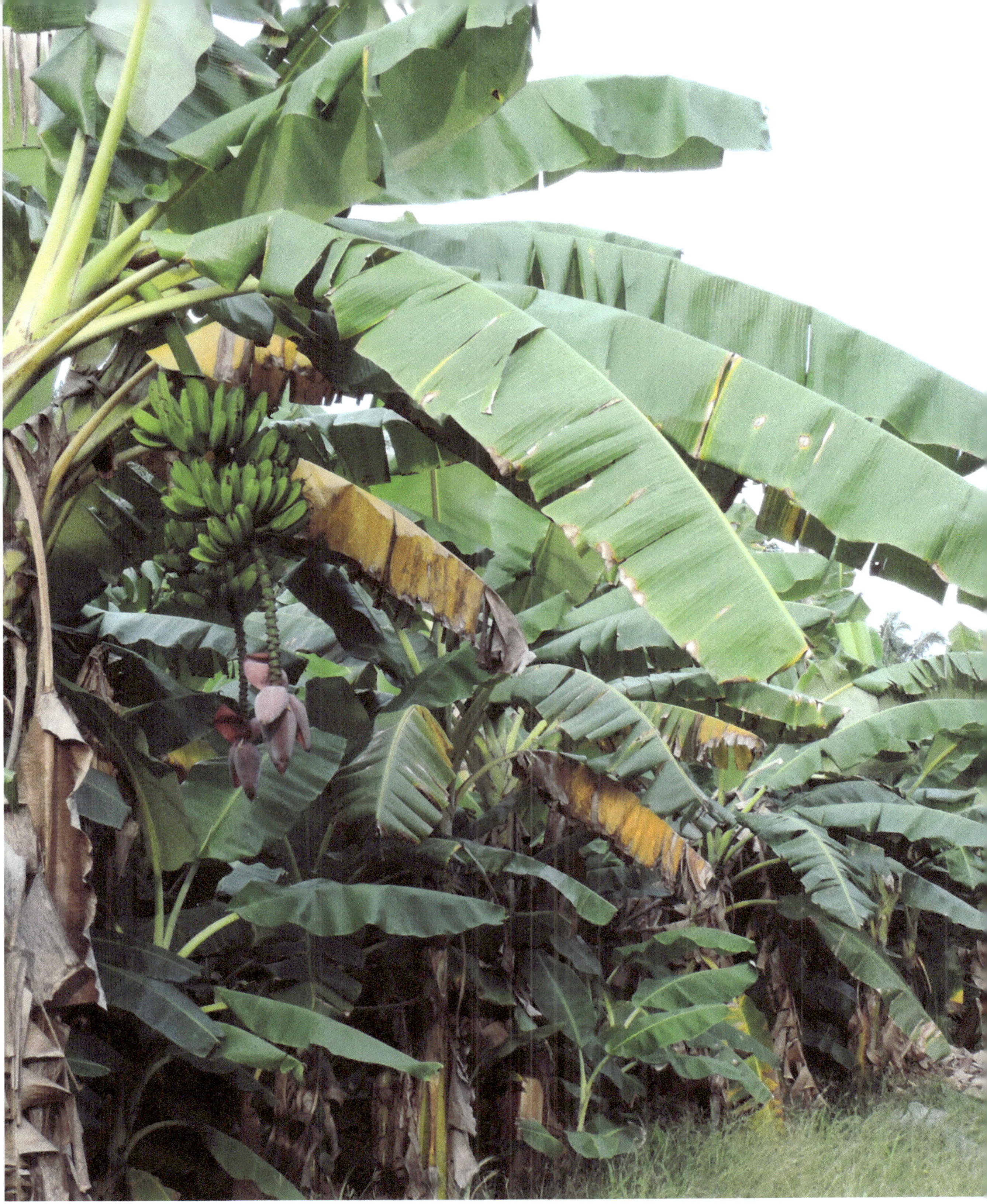

Flaming Bananas Foster

10 min   2

Instructions

1. Cut bananas in quarters, lengthwise
2. Put butter and sugar into a small saucepan and cook over medium heat
3. When the butter and sugar are mixed and melted, add the banana pieces and sauté until lightly browned
4. Sprinkle with cinnamon and remove from heat
5. Add rum and carefully light the sauce on fire, spooning it over the bananas with a long spoon until the flame is extinguished
6. Serve over ice cream, or for a shared dish, put the pan on a hot pad and scoop some ice cream into the middle

Ingredients

1	frozen banana
1 T	unsalted butter
2 t	raw sugar
1 1/2 oz	rum
·	pinch of cinnamon

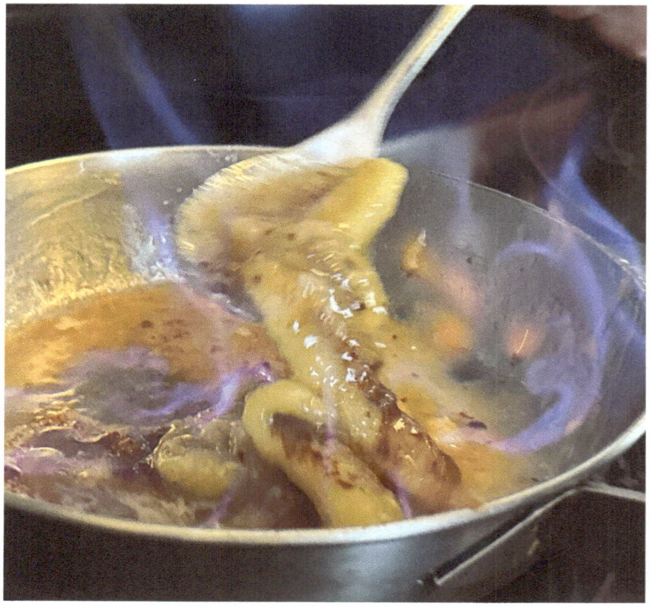

Great with coconut ice cream

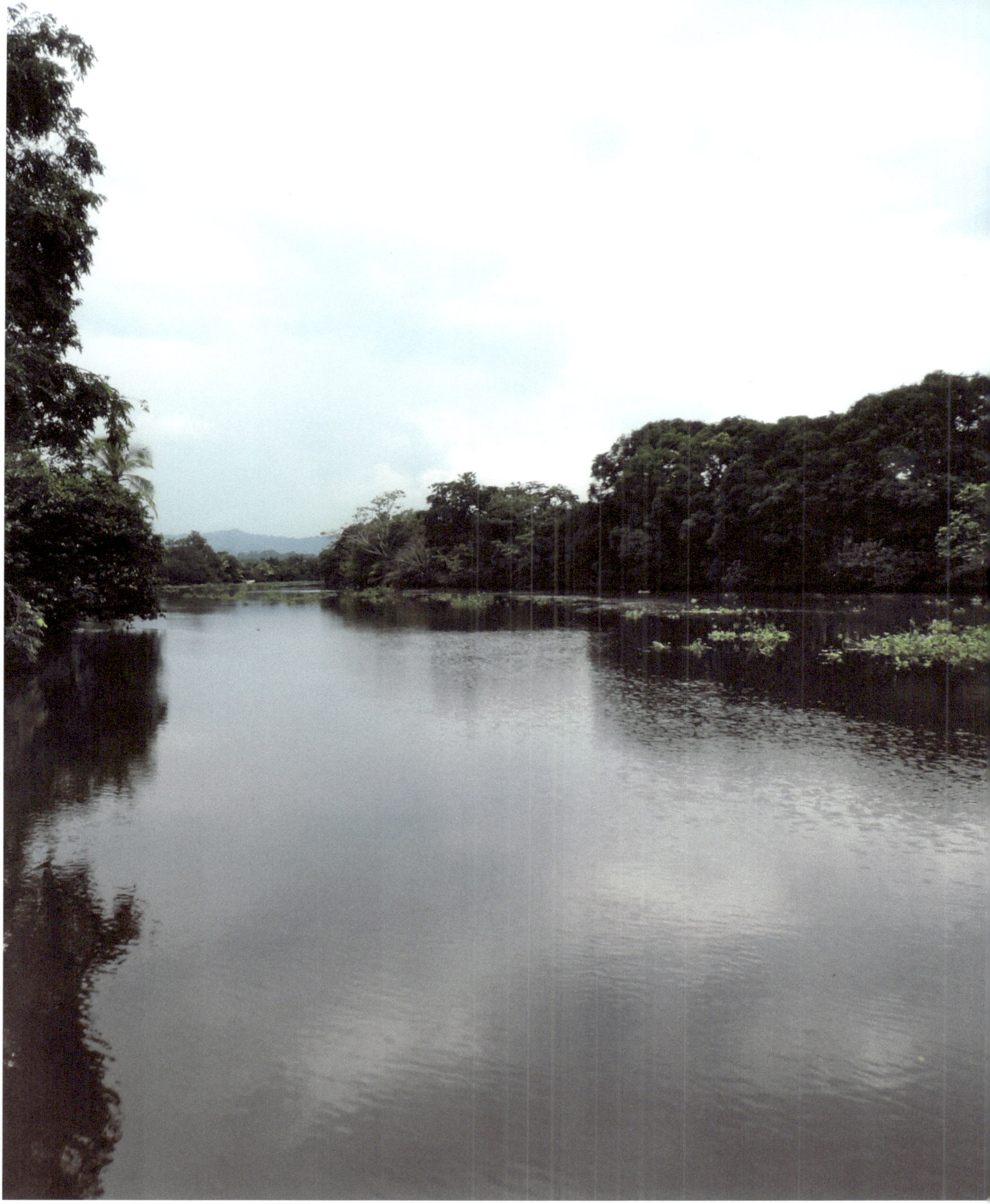

Banana Brûlée

30 min   2

Instructions

1. Mix ingredients in a blender or food processor until smooth
2. Pour batter into 4 oz porcelain ramekin bowls that are lightly greased with butter
3. Bake at 350 °F in preheated oven for 25 min
4. Sprinkle 1 t of sugar on each
5. Broil on high for 5 minutes or until sugar melts and starts to brown. Check often
6. Let cool and serve

Ingredients

3	frozen bananas
2	eggs
1/2 c	heavy cream
1 T	maple syrup
1 T	all-purpose flour
4t	raw sugar
1/2 t	vanilla extract
1/4 t	salt

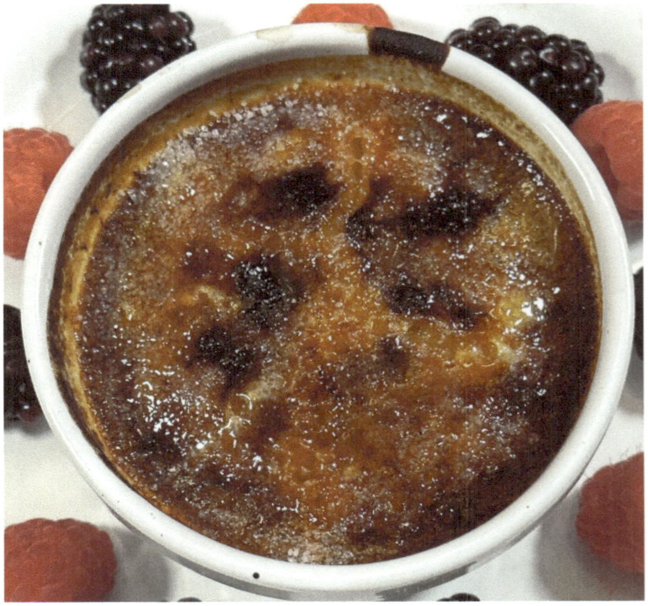

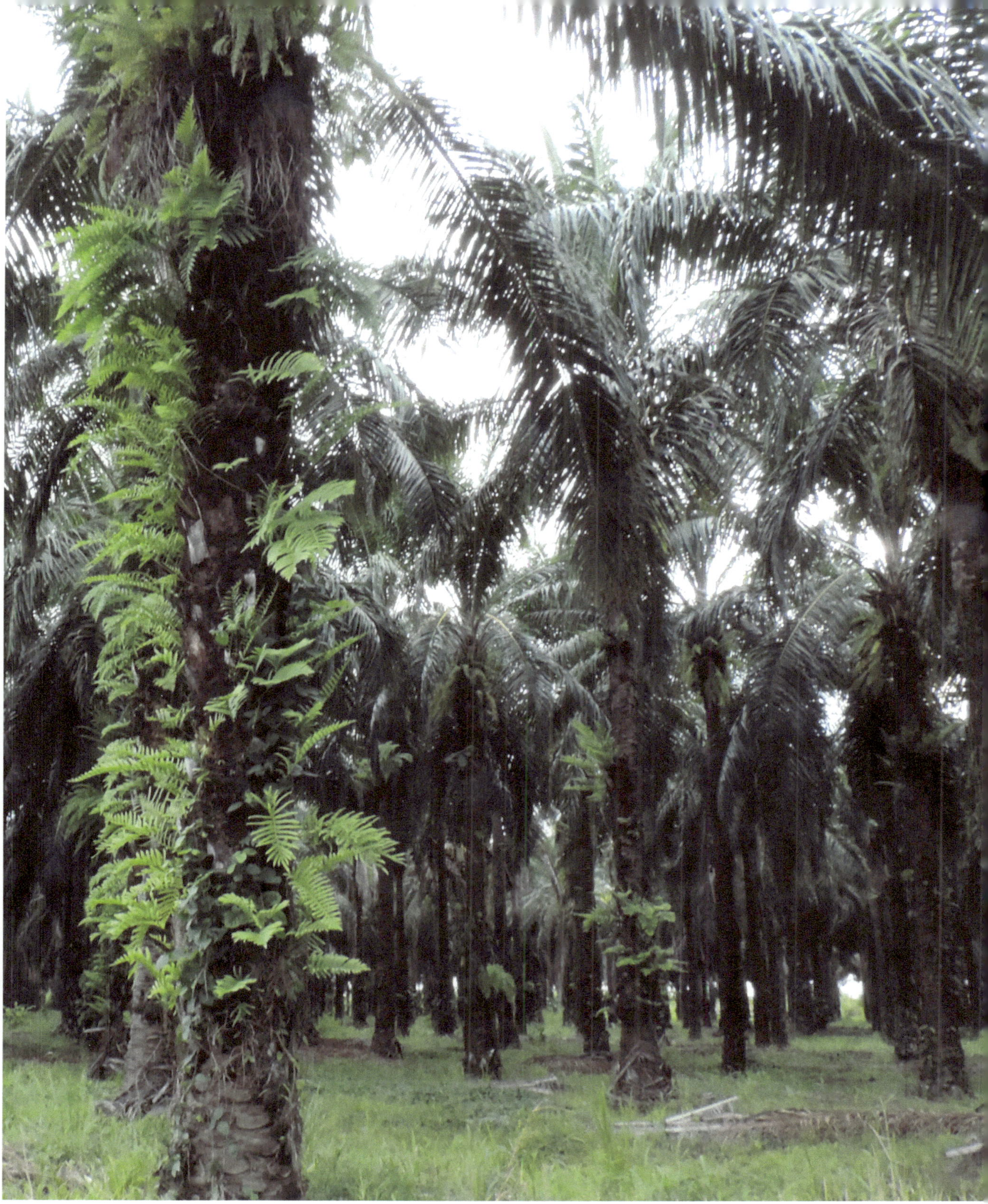

Banana Cheesecake

35 min 6

Instructions

1. Grind crackers in a processor or crush in a freezer bag
2. Mix in melted butter and sugar
3. Pack into a lightly greased 9" pie pan, pressing firmly, and set aside
4. Thaw frozen bananas and crush into a smooth mixture
5. Blend together the banana mixture, eggs, and block of cream cheese, using a food processor
6. Gently pour the batter into the pie pan, being careful not to disturb the crust
7. Bake at 350 °F in preheated oven for 55 min
8. Cover and cool in the refrigerator for 4 hrs before serving

Ingredients

1 3/4 c	Graham crackers
5T	unsalted butter
2T	raw sugar (crust)
2	frozen bananas
8oz	block cream cheese
1 c	whole milk greek yogurt
1/2 c	raw sugar (filling)
3	eggs
1 t	vanilla extract
1/4 t	salt

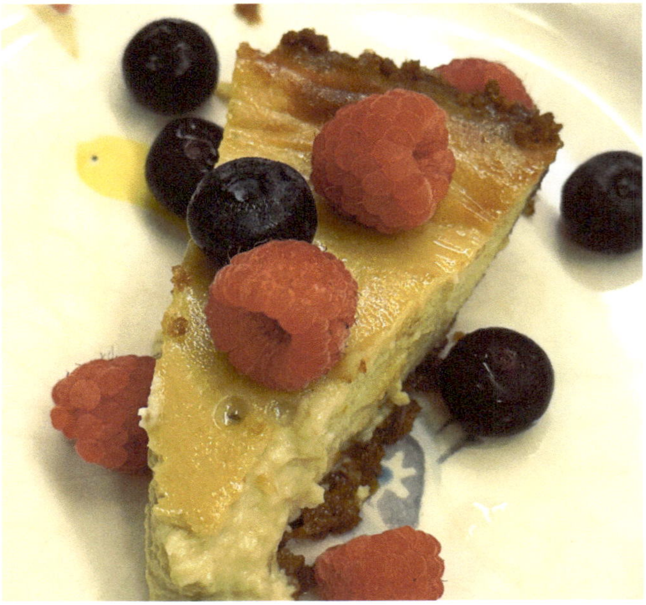

Scrumptious fresh and cold with fruit

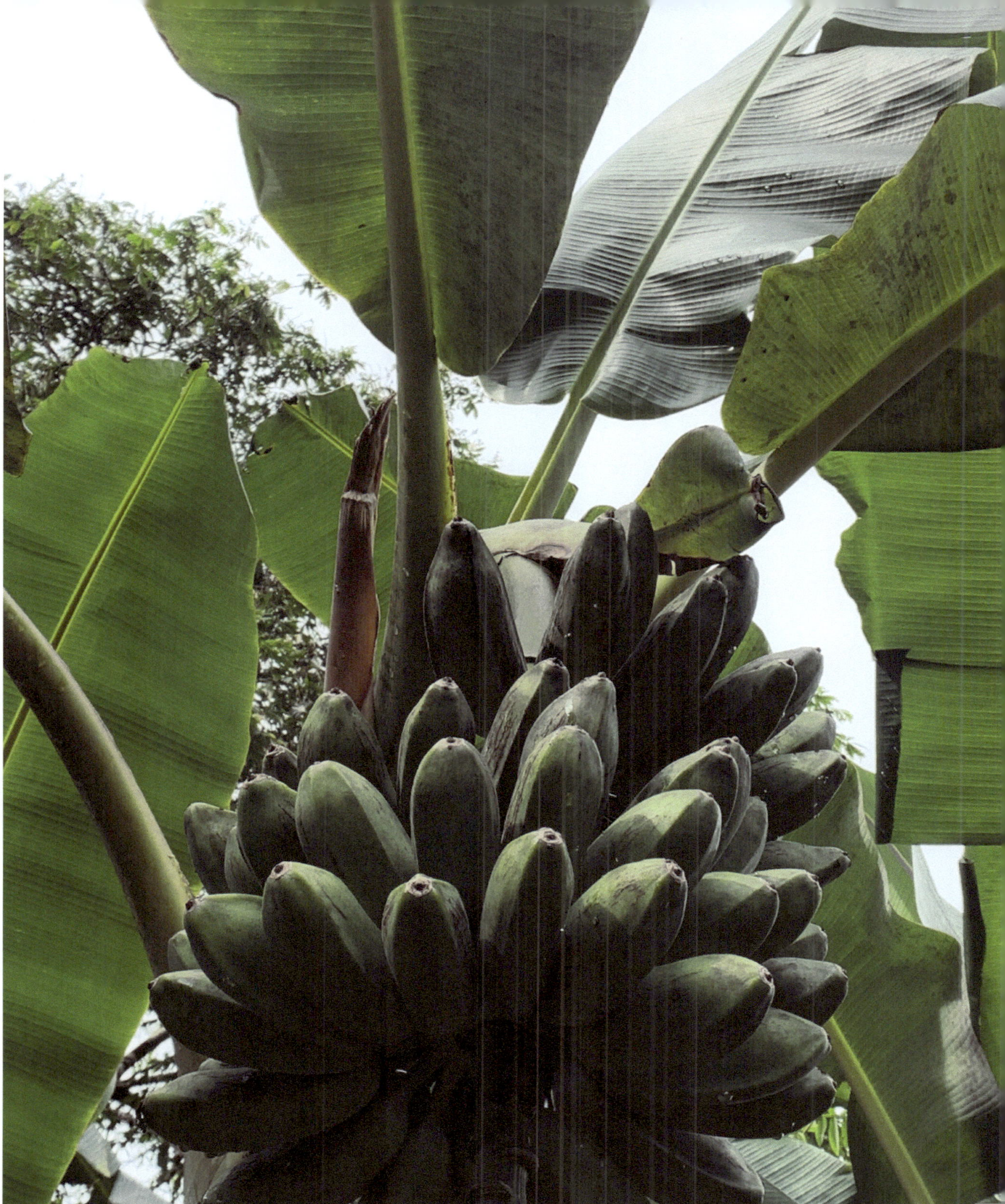

Chocolate Banana Fondue

30 min 6

Instructions

1. Defrost and mash bananas until smooth
2. Stir all ingredients in a sauce pan under very low heat until the chocolate is melted and the mixture is smooth
3. Transfer to a fondue pot and serve with strawberries, pieces of apple, and other fruit of your choice

Ingredients

2	frozen bananas
8oz	your favorite dark chocolate bar
1/2 c	half & half
1 t	vanilla extract

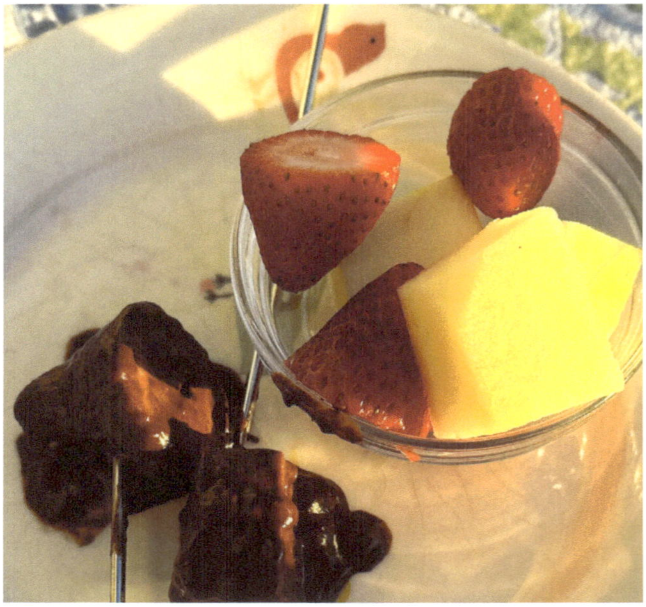

 Velvety smooth and delicious!

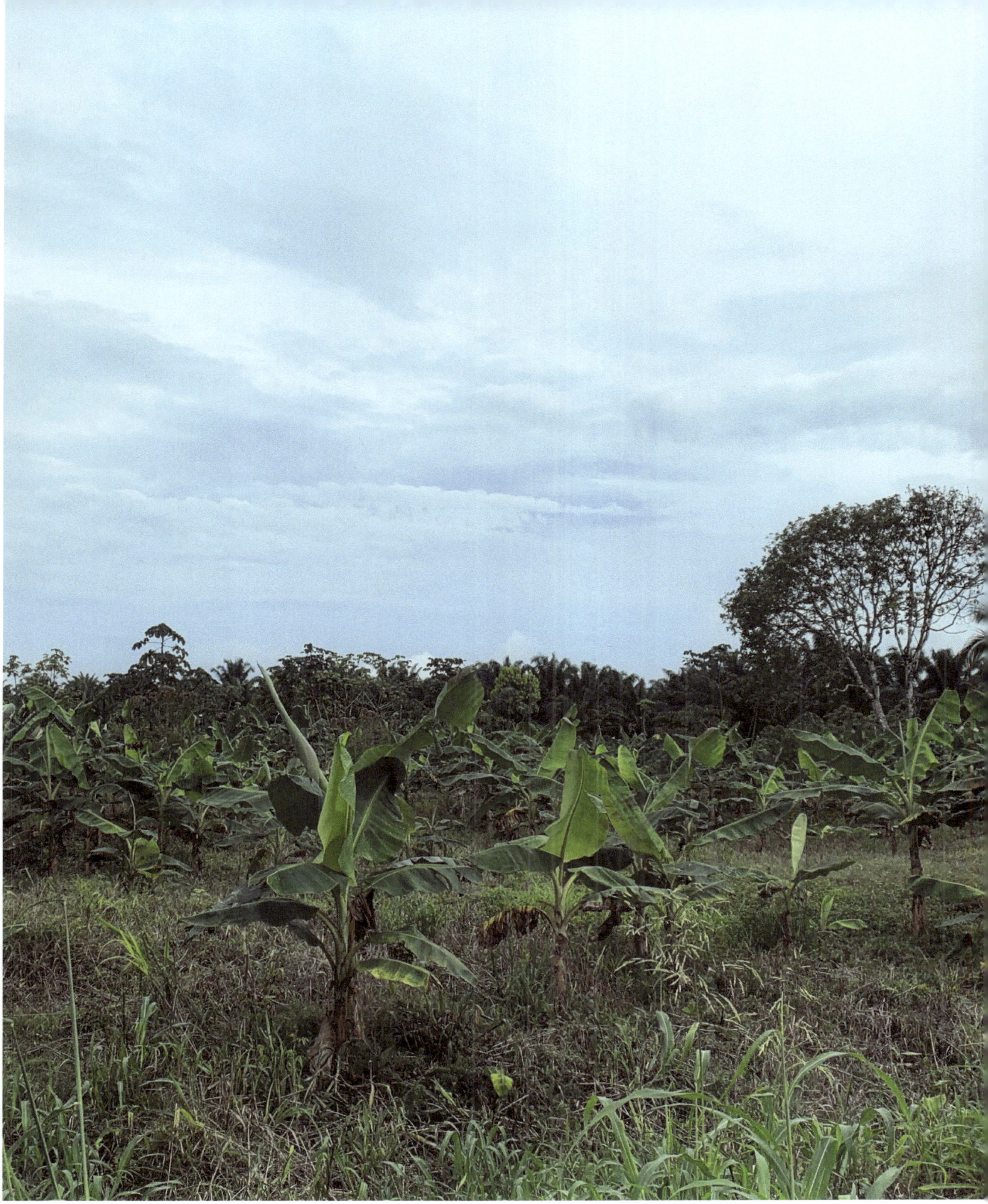

Banana Bread Pudding

30 min   2

Instructions

1. Other than the bananas and bread, mix all ingredients together
2. Cut bananas into quarter inch slices
3. Pour batter into a lightly greased 8" x 8" baking pan (or something else)
4. Bake at 350 °F for about 4 min
5. Let cool and serve

Ingredients

3	frozen bananas
2 c	bread pieces
3	eggs
1 c	whole milk
1/4 c	dried blueberries
1/4 c	raw sugar
1 T	unsalted butter
1 t	ground cinnamon
1 t	vanilla extract

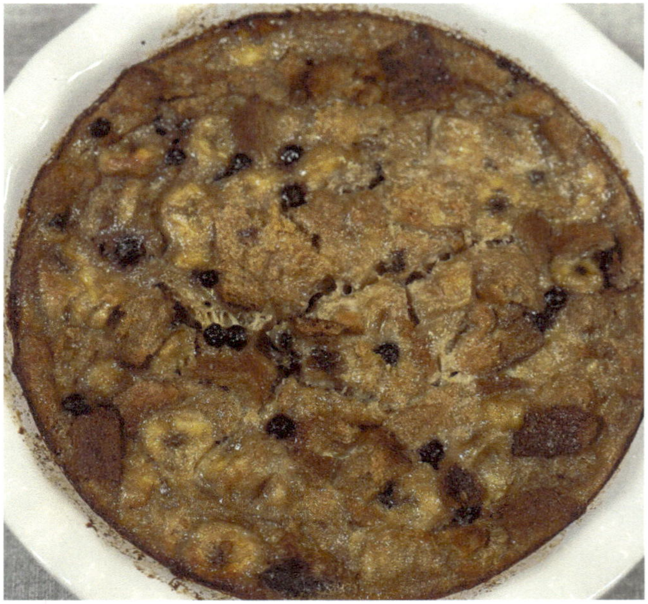

Great way to use day-old bread!

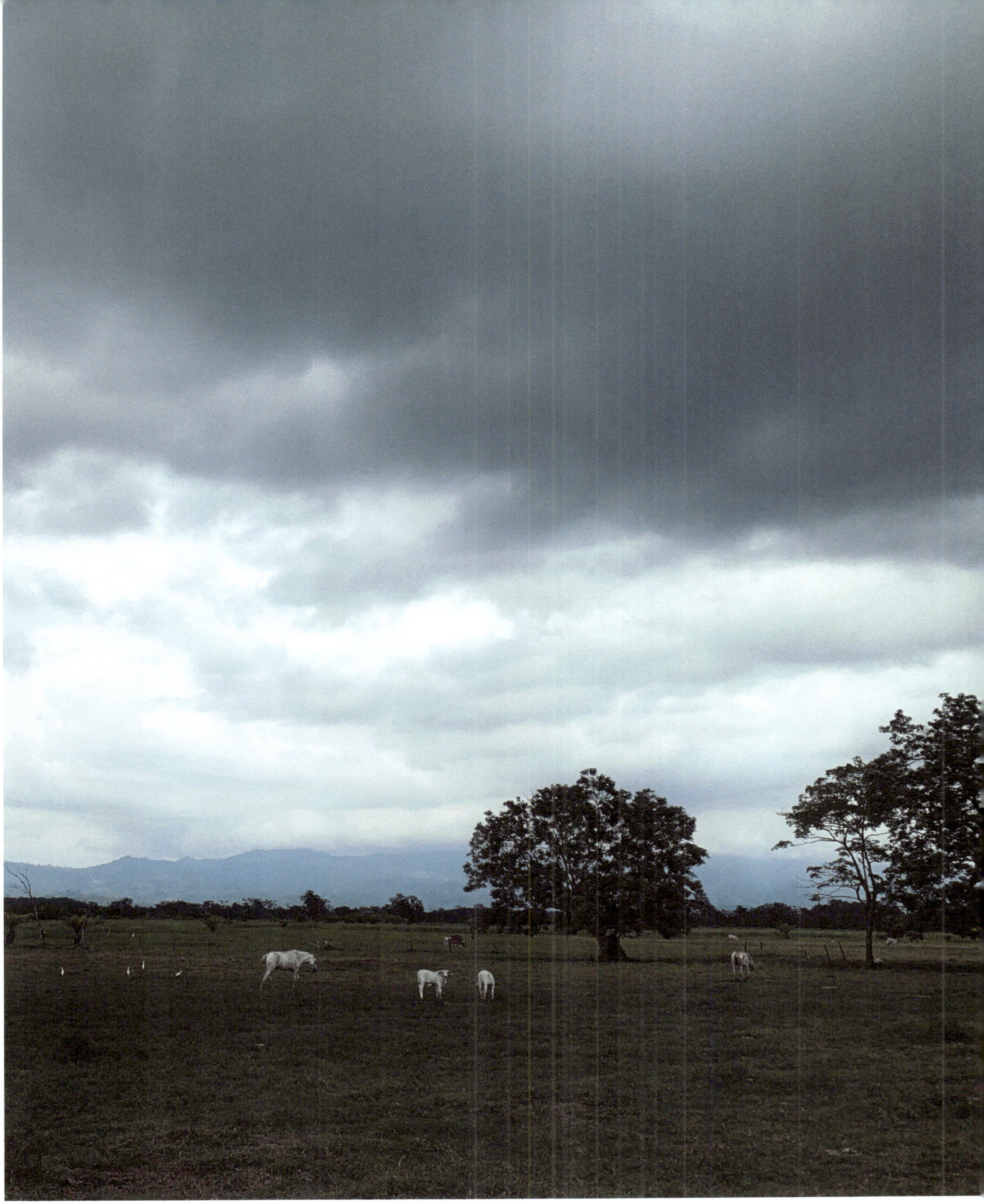

Chocolate Banana Fudge

30 min 8

Instructions

1 Thaw frozen bananas and mash into a smooth mixture

2 Melt butter in a small pan, add the banana, bring to a simmer, then immediately turn down the heat to just above low

3 Stir continuously for about 10 min

4 Add the remaining ingredients while stirring, so it doesn't clump

5 Once the chocolate is melted and all is mixed, remove from the heat and transfer to a 8" x 8" baking dish lined with parchment paper

6 When it's cool enough, chill in the fridge for at least 3 hrs before cutting and serving

Ingredients

2	frozen bananas
1 c	semi-sweet chocolate chips
1/4 c	chopped walnuts
1 T	unsalted butter
1 T	all purpose flour
1/4 t	vanilla extract

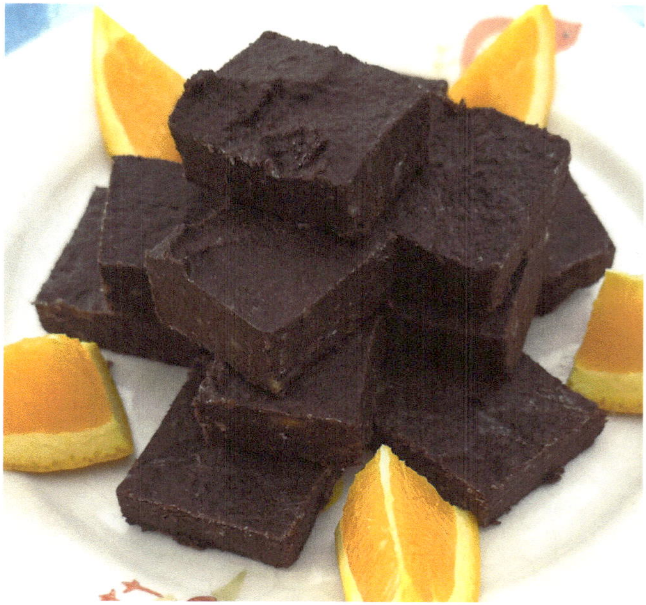

Perfect morning treat with strong dark coffee

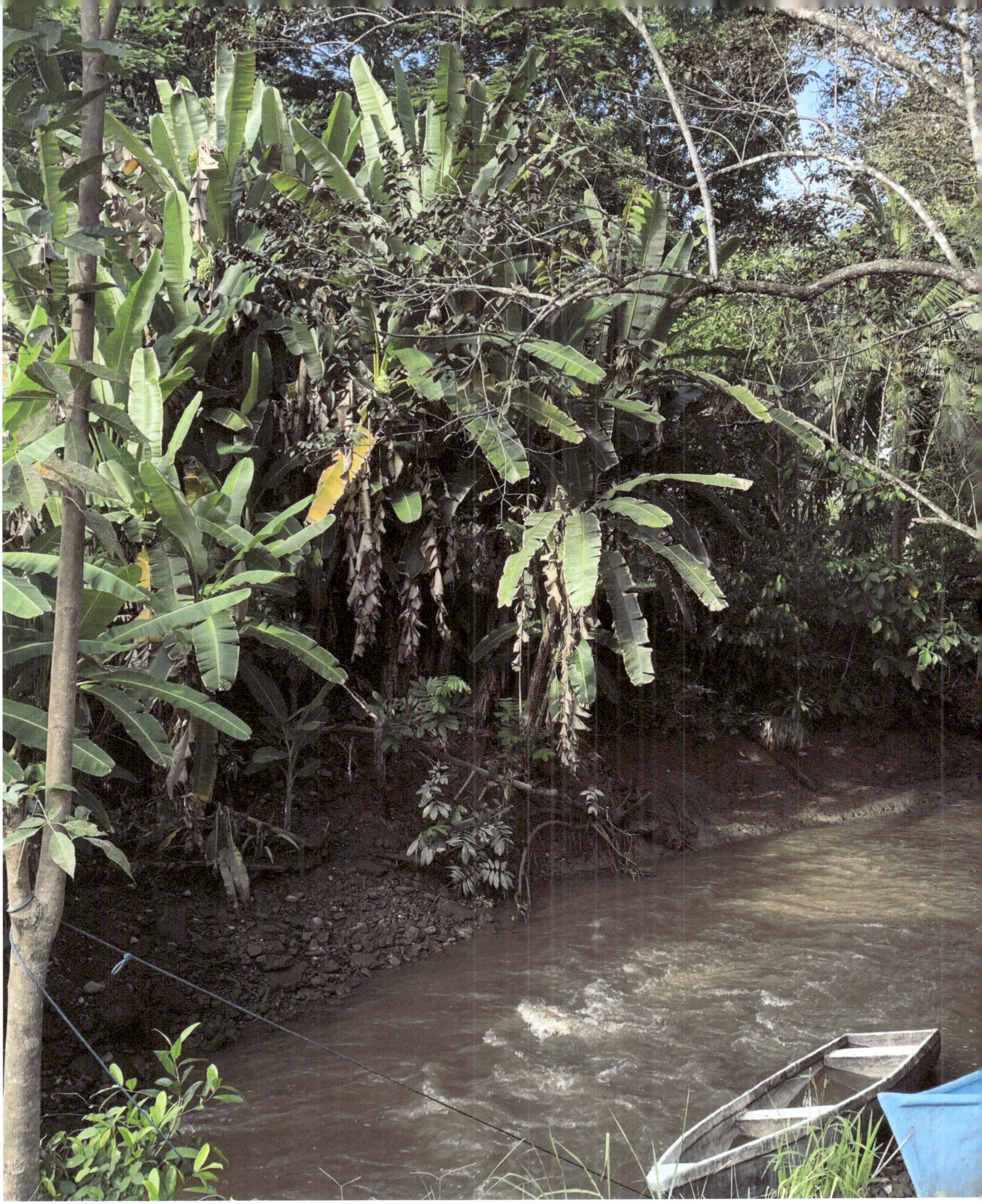

Banana Chocolate Chip Cookies

35 min 5

Instructions

1. Thaw frozen bananas and crush into a smooth mixture
2. Mix all ingredients together and let chill in the fridge for at least 1 hr
3. For each cookie, place about 2 T of dough a baking sheet with parchment paper, leaving about 2" between cookies
4. Sprinkle a little sugar on the top of each cookie
5. Bake at 350 °F for about 20 min or until the edges are slightly browned

Ingredients

3	frozen bananas
1	egg
5 oz	semi-sweet chocolate chips
1 c	old fashion rolled oats
1/2 c	raw sugar
1/3 c	unsalted butter
1/3 c	chopped walnuts
1 t	vanilla extract
1/2 t	salt
1/2 t	baking soda

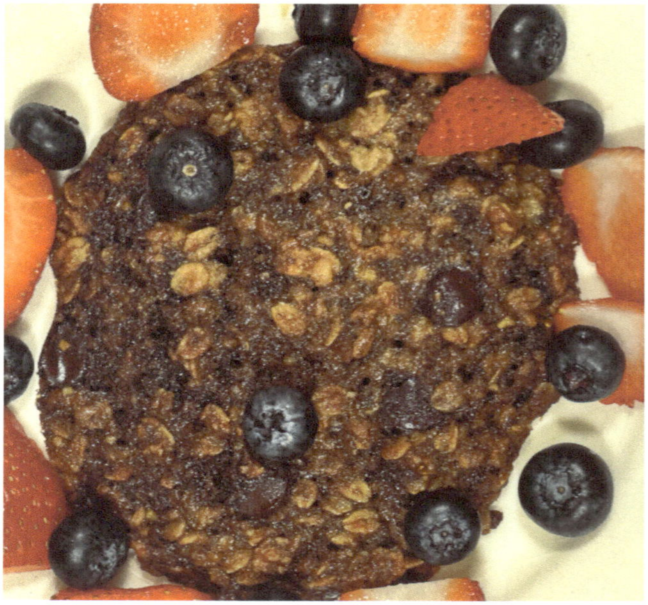

For more crunch, lower heat a little and cook longer

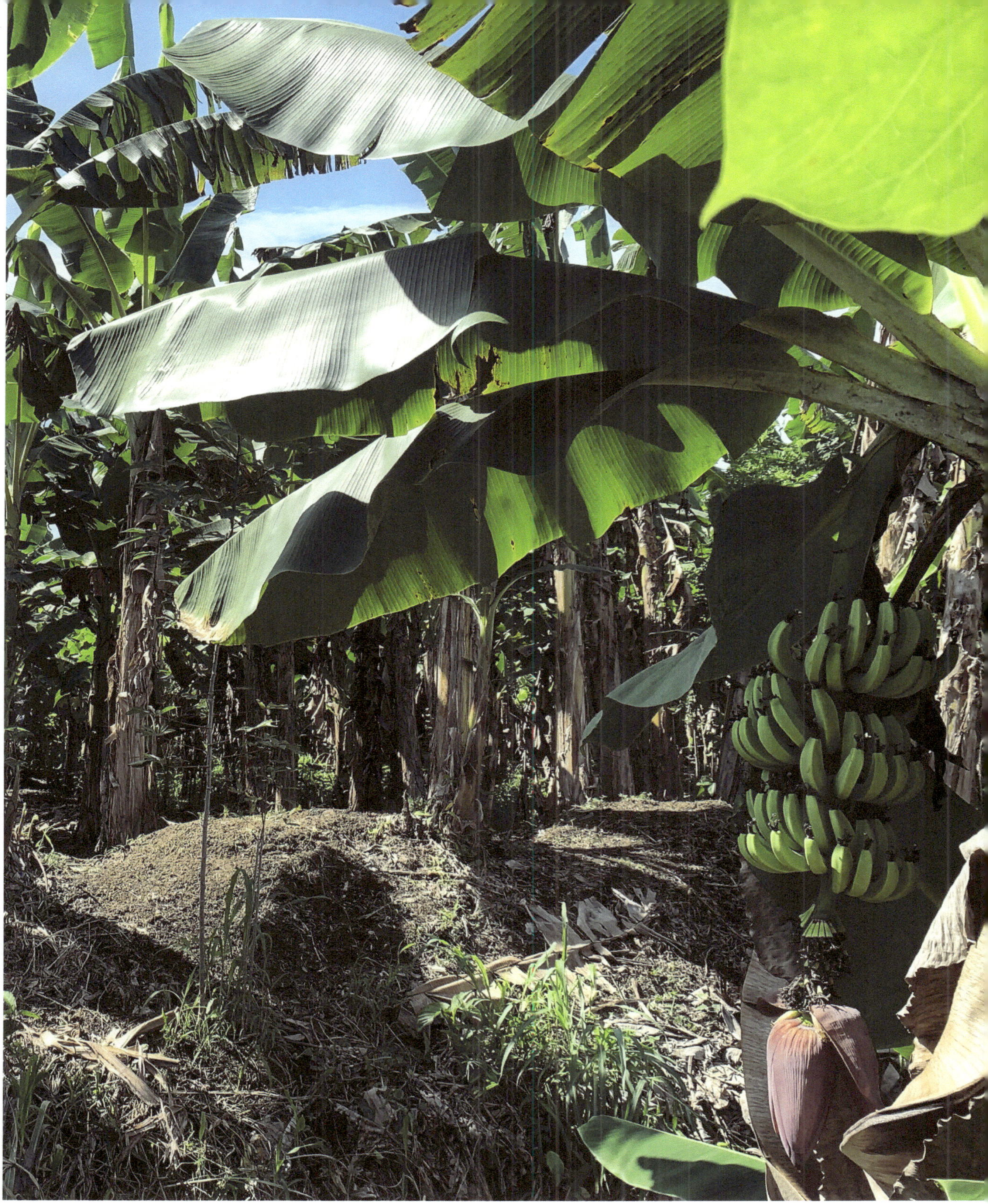

Banana Brownies

15 min 8

Instructions

1. Thaw 2 of the frozen bananas and crush into a smooth mixture
2. Mix together the wet (except the remaining 1 1/2 bananas) and dry ingredients separately then combine
3. Slice up the remaining 1 1/2 bananas and fold into the batter
4. Pour into 8" x 11" pan lined with parchment paper
5. Bake at 350 °F in preheated over for 35 min, however, after 25 min sprinkle a little coconut and sugar on top
6. Let cool at room temperature for 15 min before serving

Ingredients

3 1/2	frozen bananas
2	eggs
3/4 c	unsweetened cocoa powder
3/4 c	all-purpose flour
3/4 c	raw sugar
1/2 c	unsweetened coconut flakes
1/2 c	plain yogurt
1/3 c	unsalted butter
1 t	vanilla extract
1/2 t	salt

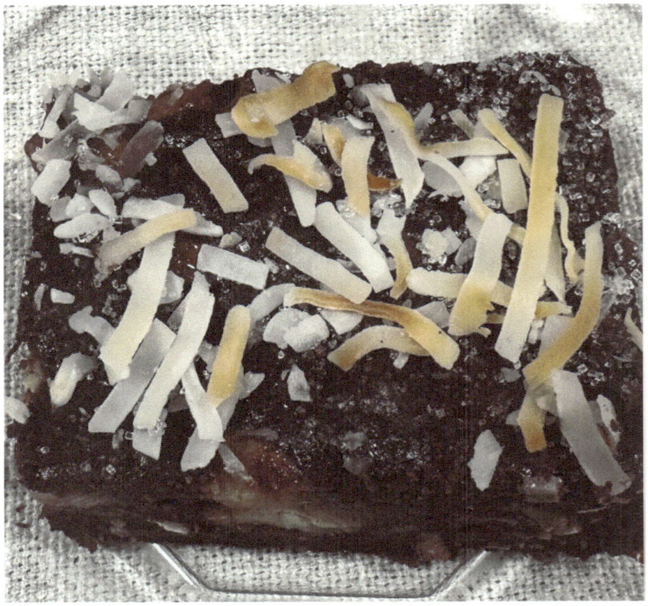

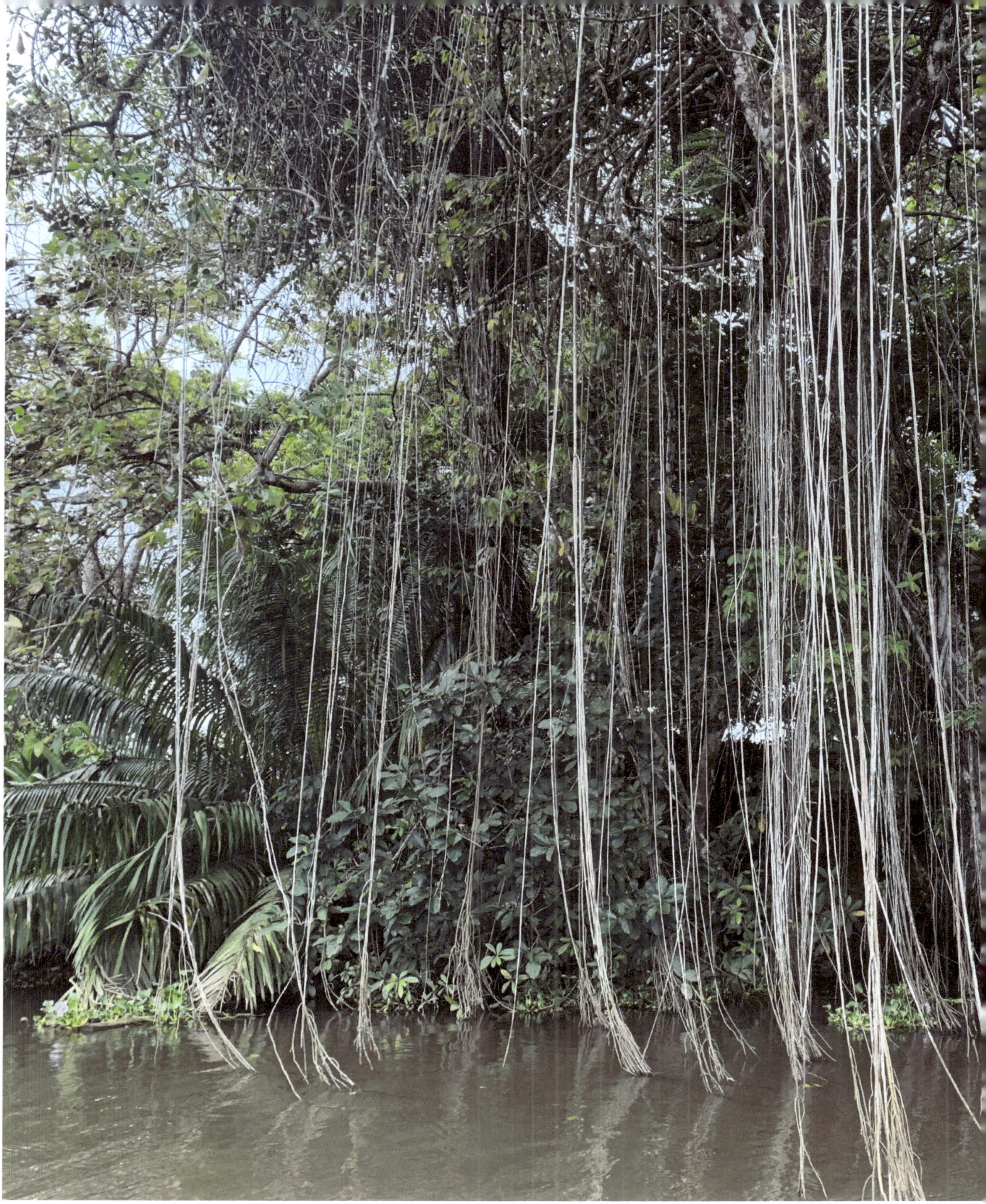

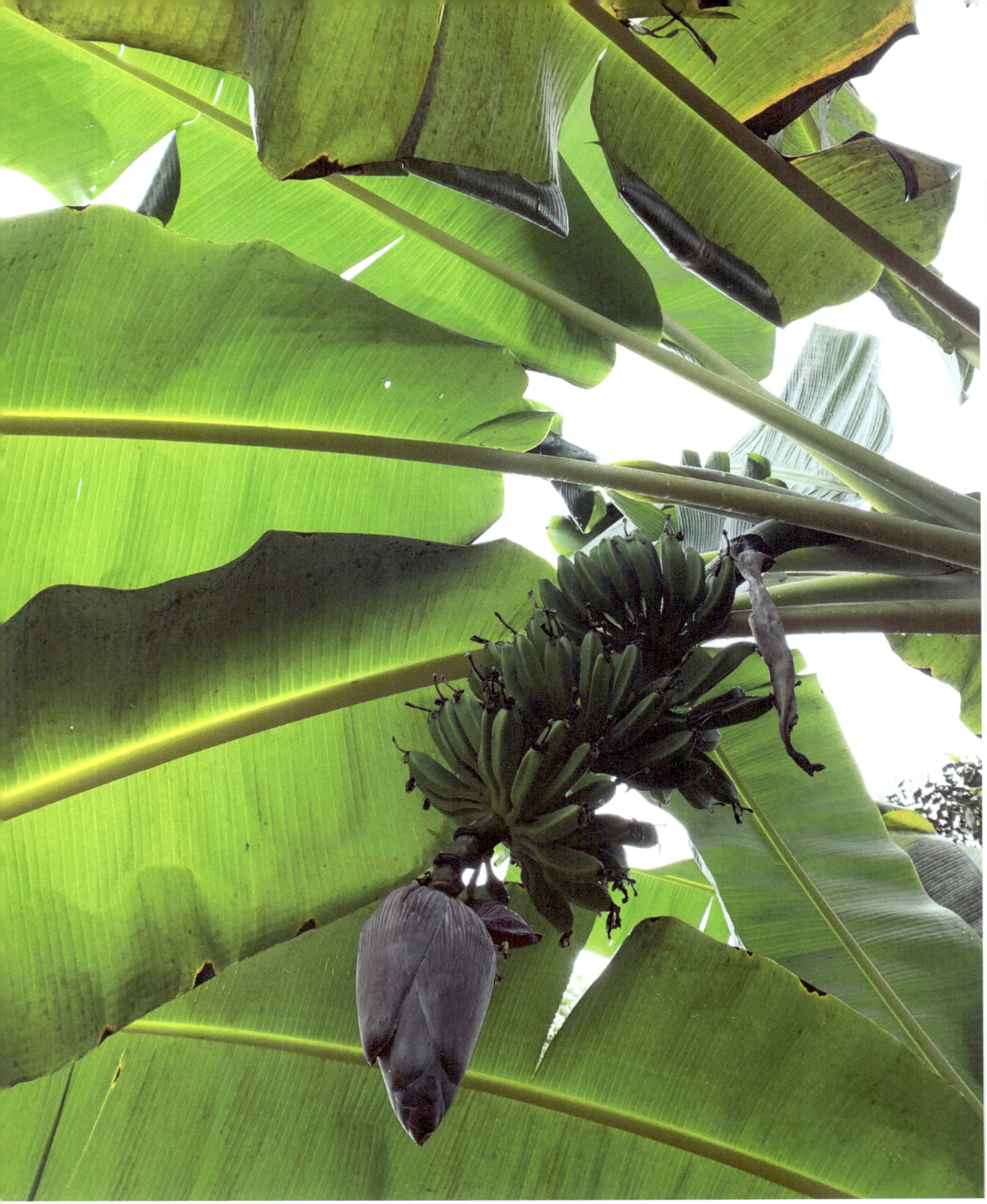

Chapter 7

Cocktails

Liqueur

20 min 10

Instructions

1 Wash the outside of the rum bottle and place upright in a medium size bowl

2 Quarter the bananas, cutting the long way, so each piece becomes four strips

3 Pour the orange juice into a second bowl and put the frozen strips in the juice

4 Insert all the strips into the bottle of rum, allowing the rum to overflow and run down the outside of the bottle into the bowl

5 Replace the cap (the bottle should be completely full with no air)

6 Remove the bottle from the bowl, twirl and shake it, and make sure the banana pieces are dispersed

7 Recover the overflow rum from the bowl and set aside for later use

8 Let the bottle sit for four days or more, occasionally giving it a twirl

9 Then, pour the mixture through a screen sieve

10 Discard the pieces and strain it again but through a fine mesh sieve

11 Pour back into the bottle and add the overflow that was set aside

To clarify, let sit for several weeks

Ingredients

1 1/2	frozen bananas
2c	orange juice
750 ml	white rum (at least 40%)

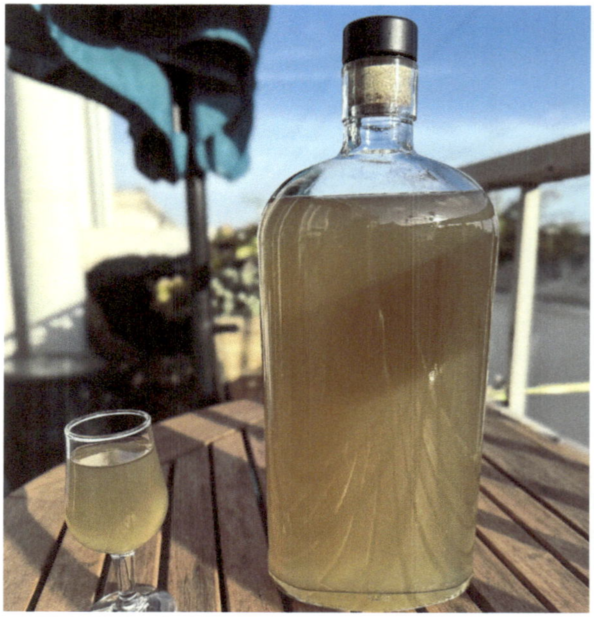

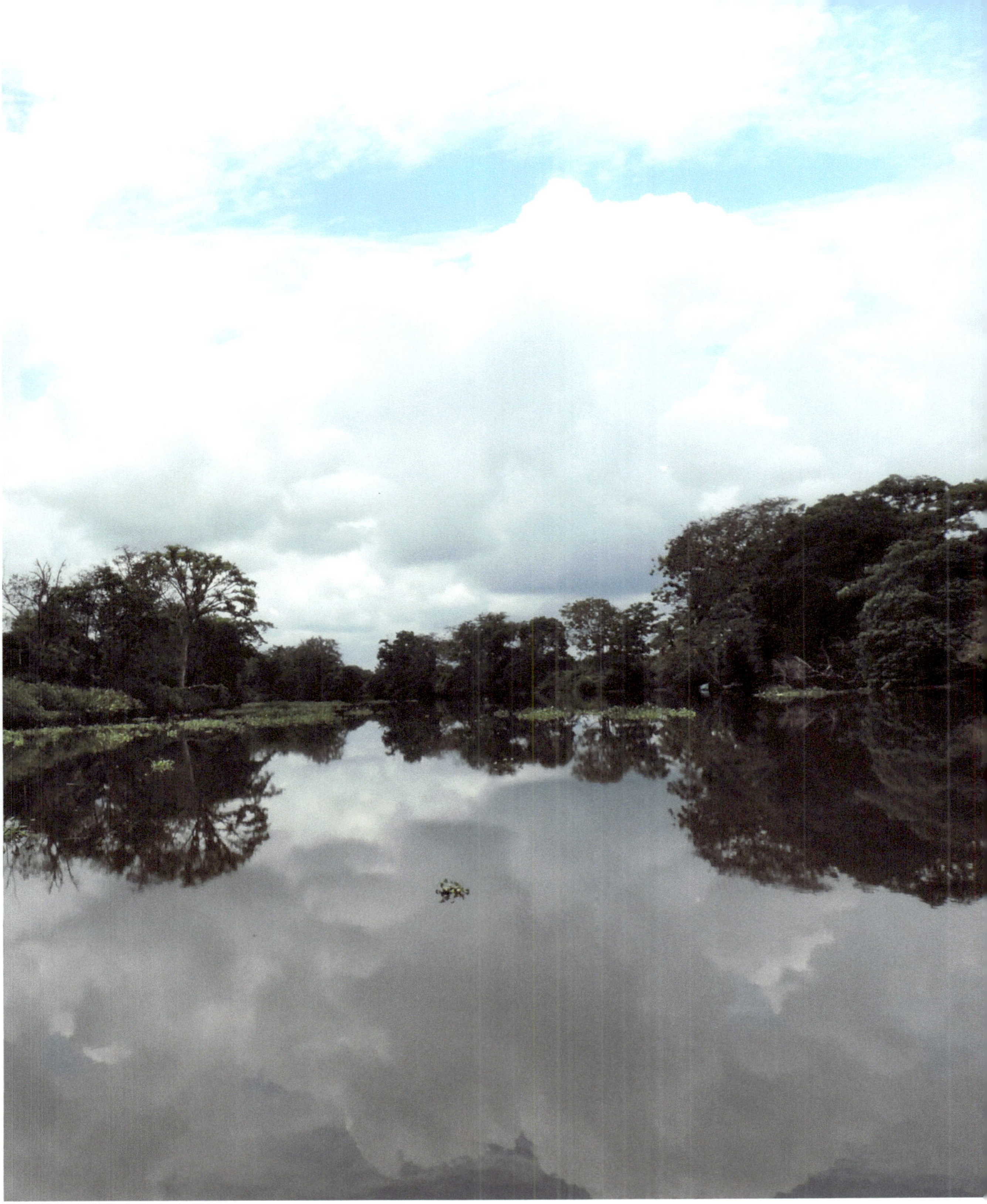

Banana Daiquiri

30 min   4

Instructions

1. Cook banana in microwave for 1 1/2 min
2. Pour the banana juice that has separated into a shaker with ice
3. Add remaining ingredients to the shaker and shake vigorously
4. Strain into a chilled class and serve with a lime twist (or wedge)

Ingredients

1	frozen banana
2 oz	white rum
	juice from 1/2 small lime
1 t	turbinado sugar

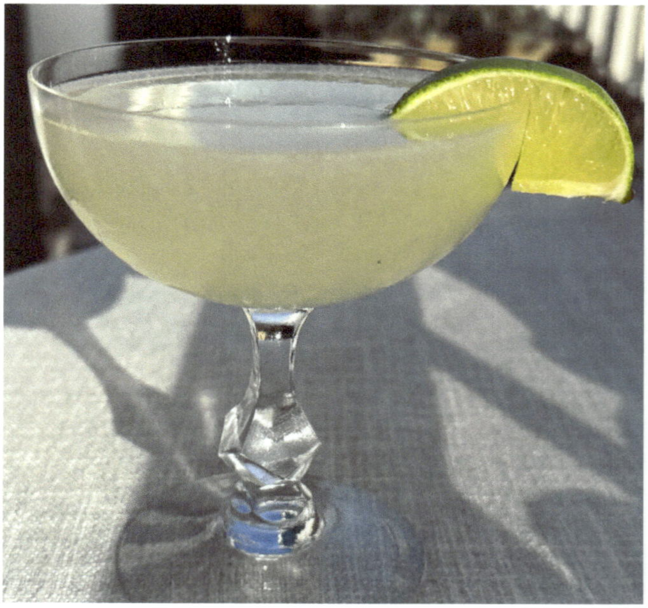

 Nice in summer at 5 pm

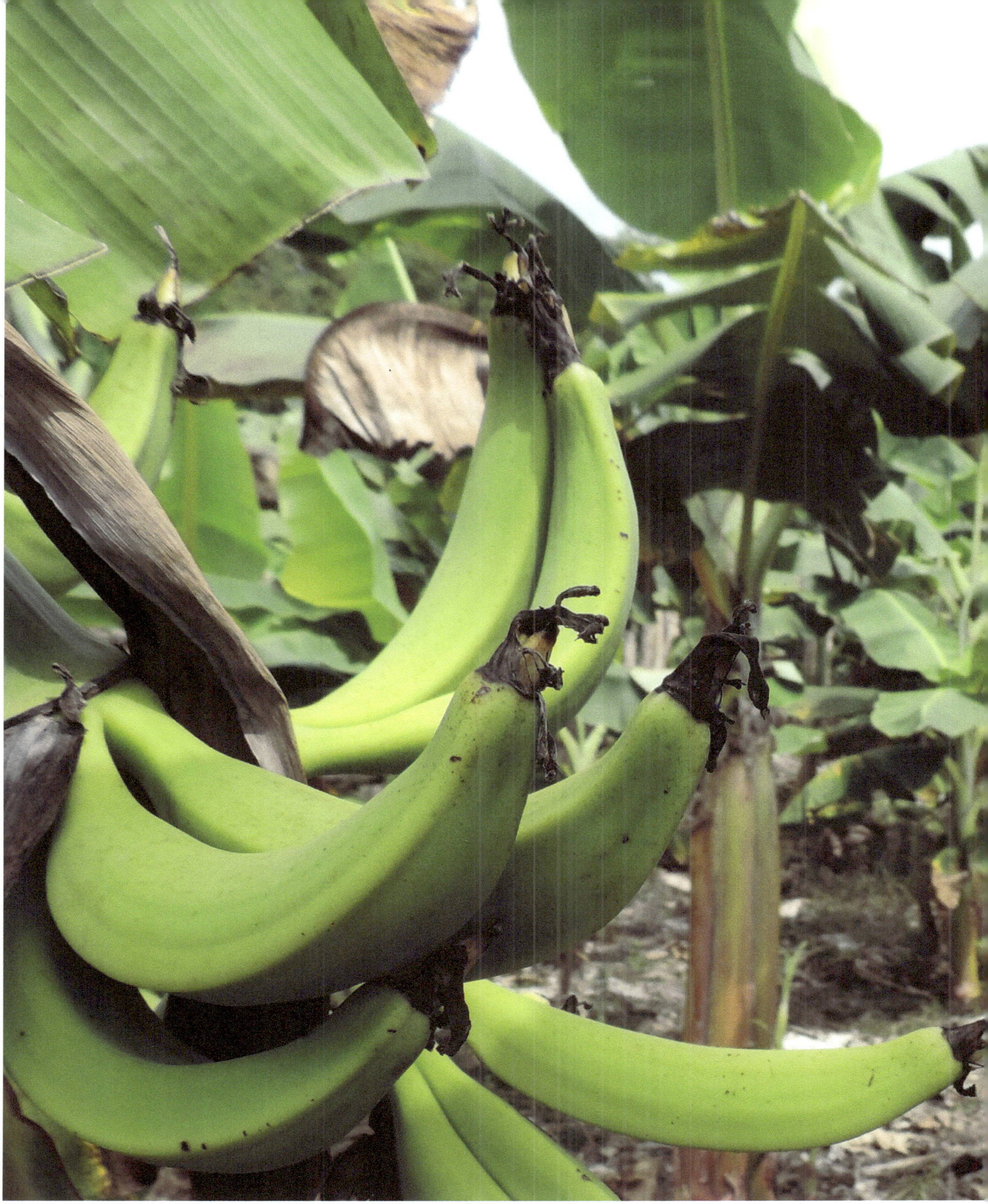

Banhattan

5 min 1

Instructions

1. Cook banana in microwave for 1 1/2 min
2. Pour the banana juice into a shaker with ice
3. Add the remaining liquid ingredients to the shaker and shake vigorously
4. Strain into a chilled class and serve with the cherry and a slice of orange

Ingredients

1	Banana
2 oz	Bourbon
1/2 oz	Vermouth (sweet, not dry)
5	Drops of bitters
·	Maraschino cherry (the wholesome kind)
2t	maraschino cherry juice
·	slice of orange

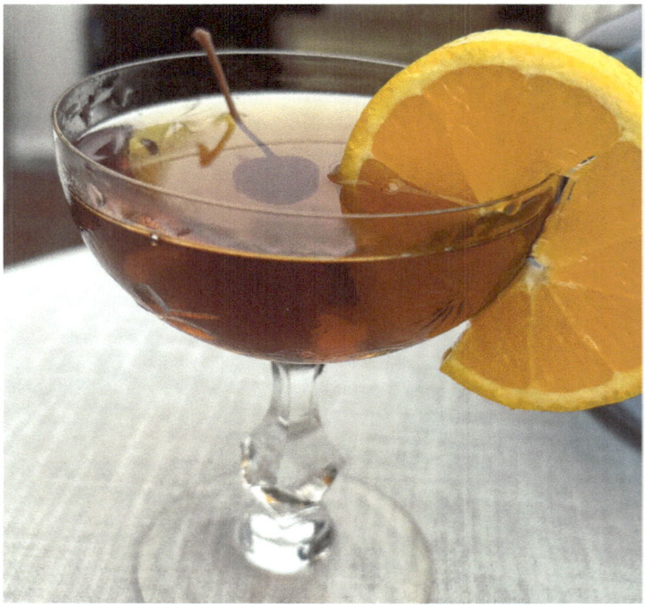

In the picture: banana liqueur was used instead of banana juice

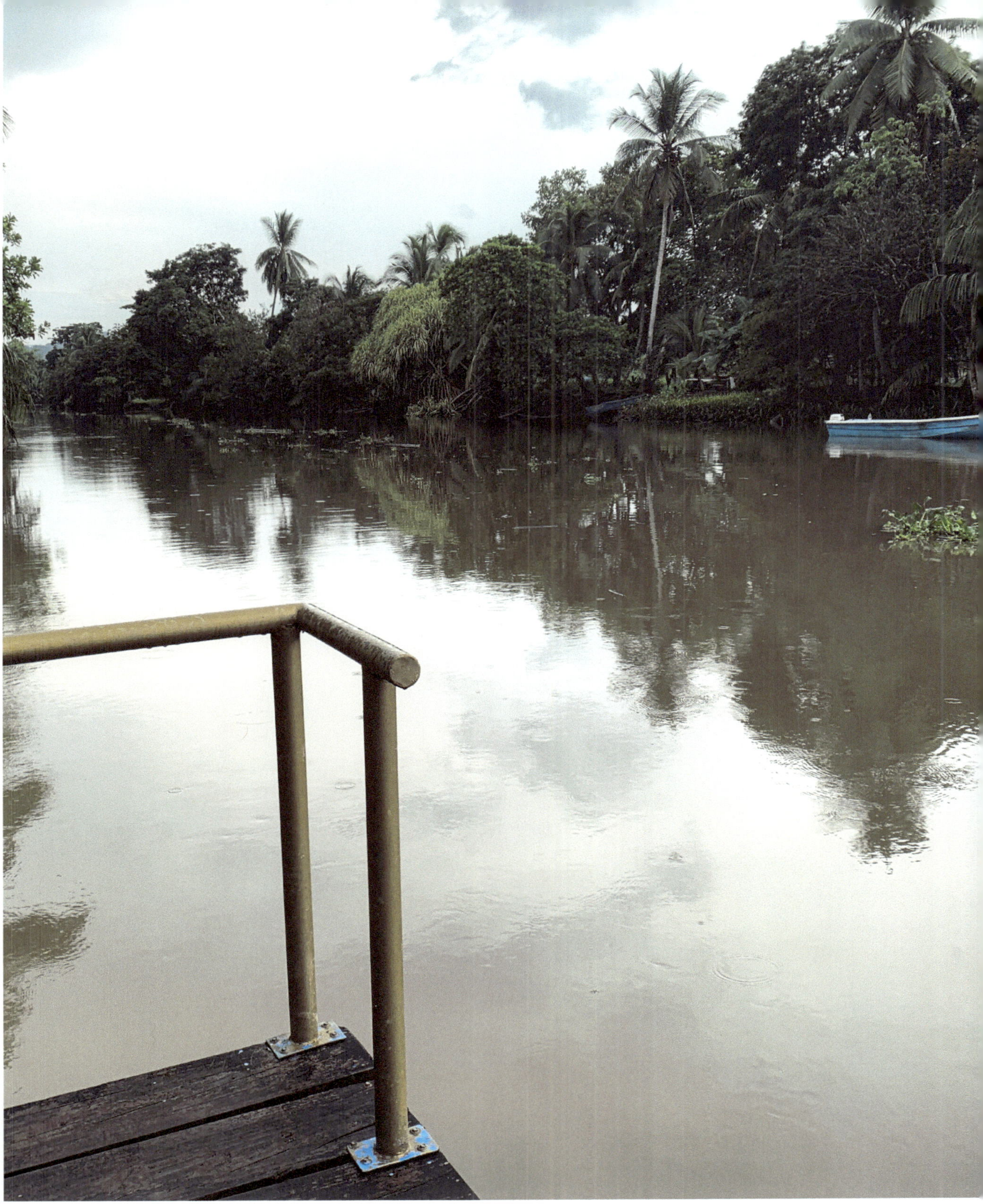

Banigni

5 min 1

Instructions

1. Cook banana in a microwave for 1 1/2
2. Pour the banana juice into a shaker with ice
3. Add the remaining liquid ingredients to the shaker and shake vigorously
4. Strain into a chilled martini class and serve with the lemon twist

Ingredients

1	frozen banana
2oz	vodka
1/2 oz	dry vermouth
	lemon twist

Dedicated to Roberto Benigni
funniest man on Earth

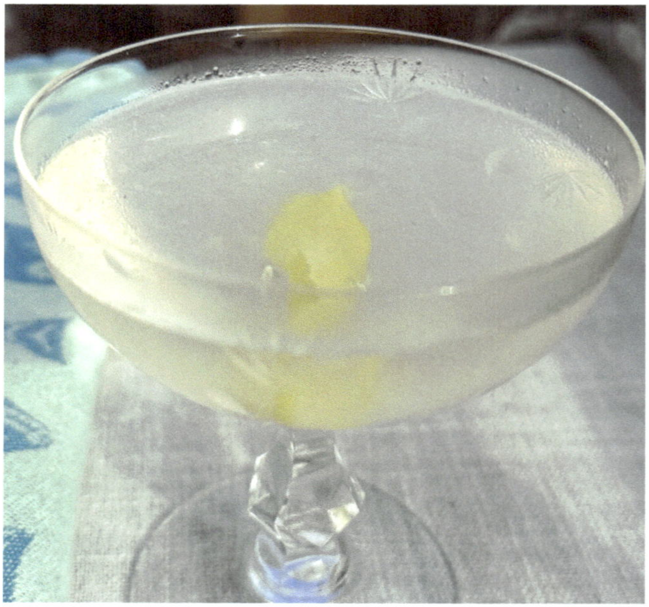

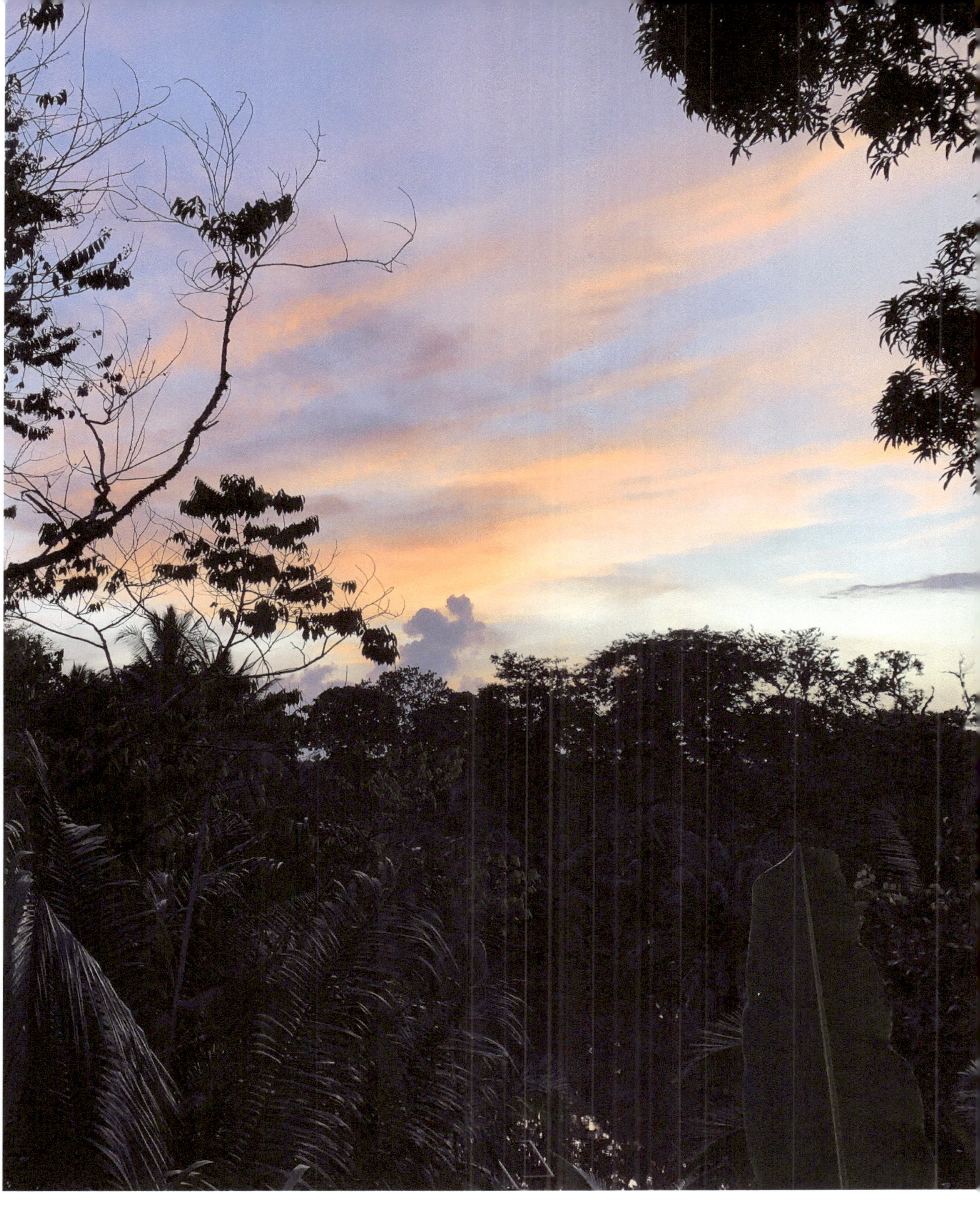

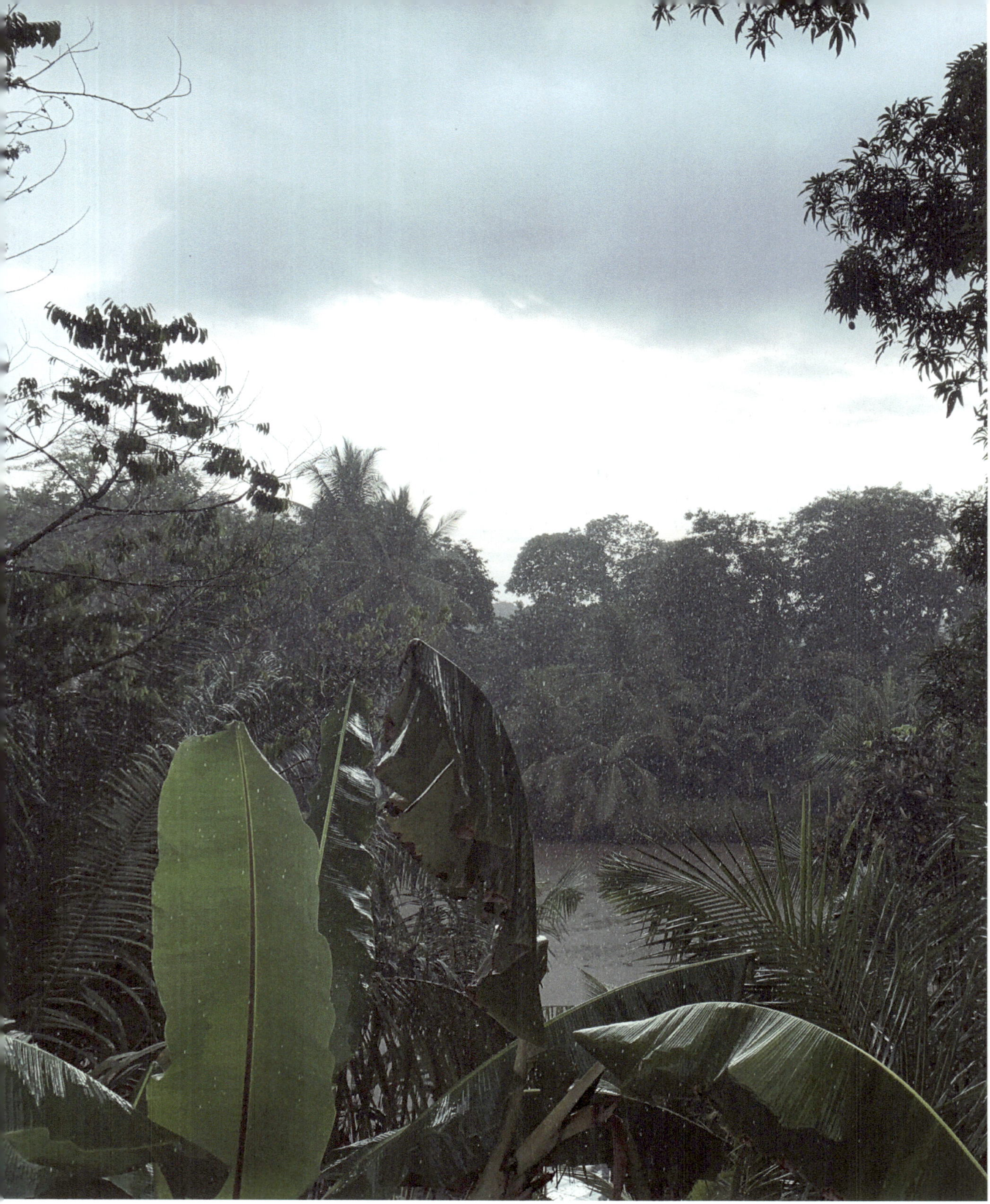

Index

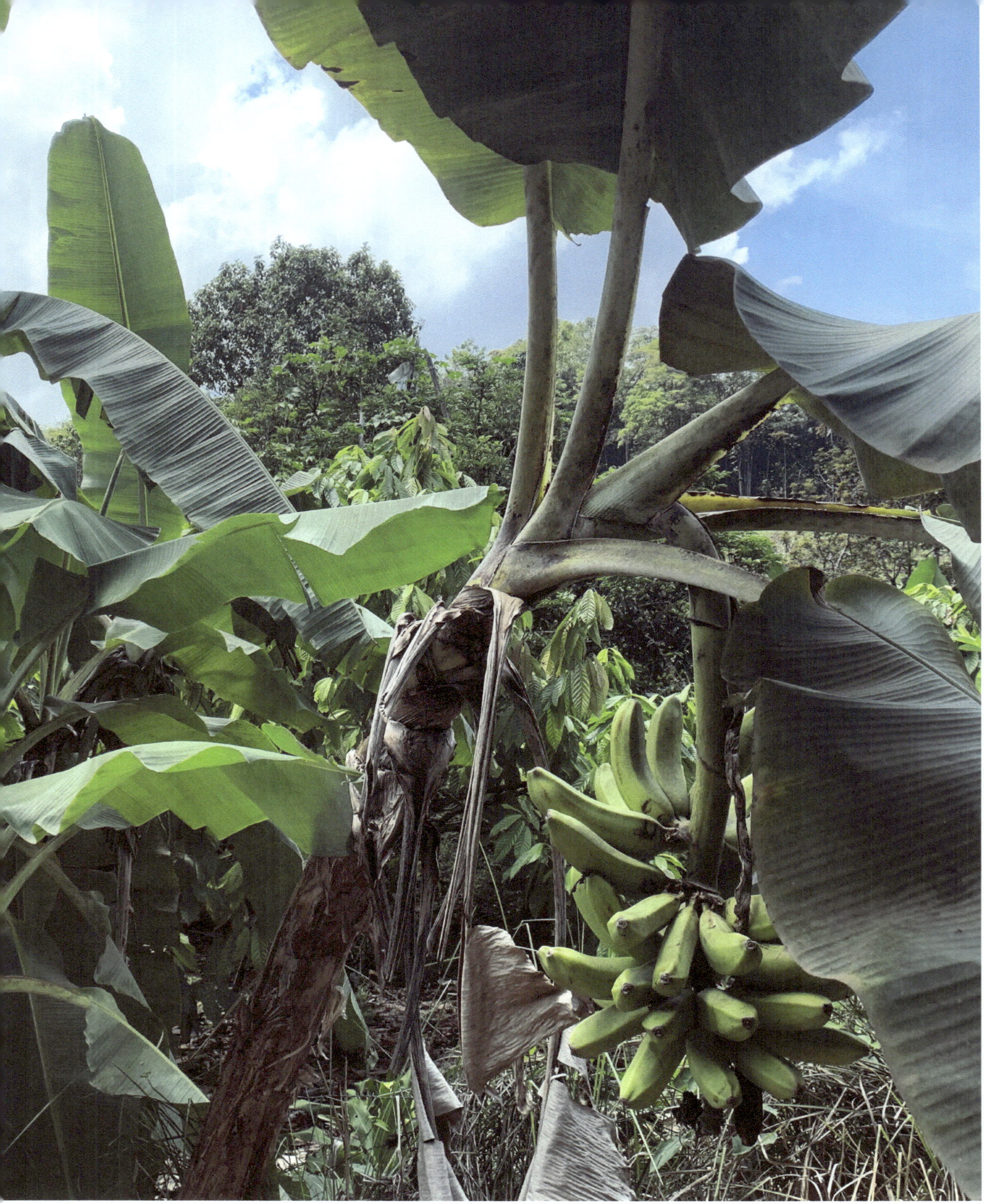

Bibliography

[1] D Gunders. 5 billion bananas get thrown away each year how reducing food waste can help solve the climate crisis. *Chicago Tribune; Opinion; April 9*, 1995.

[2] J Keus. The sad story of the rejected bananas used as cattle feed: a study in the atlantic zone of costa rica. *Report-Atlantic Zone Programme/CATIE-AUW-MAG; number 95*, 1995.

[3] Sidonia Martínez, Andreina Roman-Chipantiza, Asma Boubertakh, and Javier Carballo. Banana drying: A review on methods and advances. *Food Reviews International*, pages 1–39, 2023.

www.ingramcontent.com/pod-product-compliance
Ingram Content Group UK Ltd.
Pitfield, Milton Keynes, MK11 3LW, UK
UKHW060010051026
15591UKWH00002B/131
* 9 7 8 1 9 3 9 9 8 6 6 4 1 *